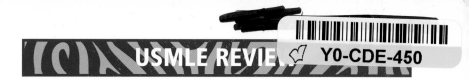
DERMATOLOGY
for the
Boards and Wards

Other books in the Boards and Wards series:
Boards & Wards — USMLE Steps 2 and 3
Pathophysiology for the Boards & Wards — USMLE Step 1
Immunology for the Boards & Wards — USMLE Step 1
Microbiology for the Boards & Wards — USMLE Step 1
Ophthalmology/ENT for the Boards & Wards — USMLE Steps 1, 2, and 3
Behavioral Sciences and Outpatient Medicine for the Boards & Wards —
   USMLE Steps 1, 2, and 3

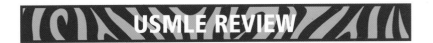
USMLE REVIEW

DERMATOLOGY
for the
Boards and Wards

Carlos Ayala, MD
Clinical Fellow in Otology and Laryngology
Harvard Medical School
Resident in Otolaryngology
Harvard Otolaryngology Residency Program
Boston, Massachussetts

Brad Spellberg, MD
Resident in Internal Medicine
Harbor-UCLA Medical Center
Torrance, California

b

**Blackwell
Science**

©2001 by Carlos Ayala and Brad Spellberg, and Blackwell Science, Inc.

BLACKWELL SCIENCE, INC.

Editorial Offices:
Commerce Place, 350 Main Street, Malden, Massachusetts 02148, USA
Osney Mead, Oxford OX2 0EL, England
25 John Street, London WC1N 2BL, England
23 Ainslie Place, Edinburgh EH3 6AJ, Scotland
54 University Street, Carlton, Victoria 3053, Australia

Other Editorial Offices:
Blackwell Wissenschafts-Verlag GmbH, Kurfürstendamm 57, 10707 Berlin, Germany
Blackwell Science KK, MG Kodenmacho Building, 7-10 Kodenmacho Nihonbashi, Chuo-ku,
   Tokyo 104, Japan
Iowa State University Press, A Blackwell Science Company, 2121 S. State Avenue, Ames,
   Iowa 50014-8300, USA

Distributors:

USA
Blackwell Science, Inc.
Commerce Place
350 Main Street
Malden, Massachusetts 02148
(Telephone orders: 800-215-1000 or
   781-388-8250; fax orders: 781-388-8270)

Canada
Login Brothers Book Company
324 Saulteaux Crescent
Winnipeg, Manitoba R3J 3T2
(Telephone orders: 204-837-2987)

Australia
Blackwell Science Pty, Ltd.
54 University Street
Carlton, Victoria 3053
(Telephone orders: 03-9347-0300;
   fax orders: 03-9349-3016)

Outside North America and Australia
Blackwell Science, Ltd.
c/o Marston Book Services, Ltd.
P.O. Box 269
Abingdon
Oxon OX14 4YN
England
(Telephone orders: 44-01235-465500;
   fax orders: 44-01235-465555)

Acquisitions: Beverly Copland
Development: Julia Casson
Production: Shawn Girsberger

Manufacturing: Lisa Flanagan
Marketing Manager: Toni Fournier
**Printed and bound by Walsworth Publishing
Company**

Printed in the United States of America
01 02 03 04 5 4 3 2 1

The Blackwell Science logo is a trade mark of Blackwell Science Ltd., registered at the United
Kingdom Trade Marks Registry

Library of Congress Cataloging-in-Publication Data
Ayala, Carlos, MD.
   Dermatology for the boards and wards / by Carlos Ayala and Brad Spellberg.
      p.; cm.
   ISBN 0-632-04572-8
   1. Dermatology—Examinations, questions, etc. I. Spellberg, Brad. II. Title.
   [DNLM: 1. Dermatology—Examination Questions. WR 18.2 A973d 2001]
   RL74.2 .A96 2001
   616.5'0076—dc21

                                                                                   2001025024

TABLE OF CONTENTS

TABLES

ABBREVIATIONS

$\rightarrow$	causes/leads to/analysis shows
$\uparrow$ / $\downarrow$	increases or high/decreases or low
$1°/2°/3°$	primary/secondary/tertiary
Dx	diagnosis
DDx	differential diagnosis
dz	disease
hr(s)	hour(s)
hx	history
mets	metastases
mo(s)	months
pt(s)	patient(s)
Px	prognosis
Si/Sx	signs/symptoms
Tx	Treatment
yr(s)	years(s)

PREFACE

The dermatology needed for the boards revolves around pattern recognition of classic physical findings. Herein we combine a concise review of testable diseases in dermatology with a series of color photographs displaying classic patterns of diseases which might be pictured on the boards. Good luck!

FIGURES

I. TERMINOLOGY

1. Macule = flat discoloration (see Fig. 1.1)

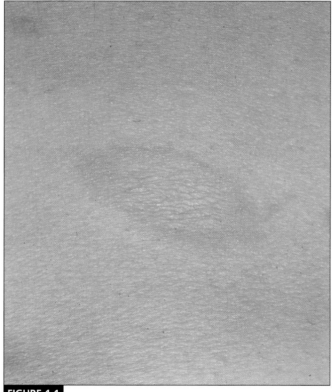

FIGURE 1.1

This erythematous macule is the typical herald patch of pityriasis rosea. (courtesy of Dr. Steven Gammer)

2. Papule = elevated skin lesion, <1 cm in diameter (see Fig. 1.2)

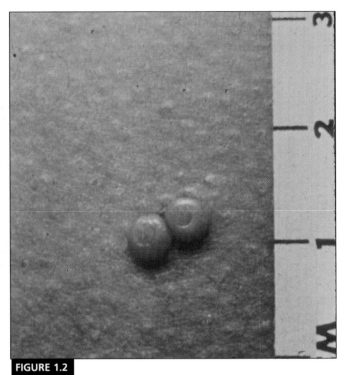

FIGURE 1.2

Molluscum contagiosum demonstrating classic papules. (courtesy of Dr. Douglas Smith)

3. Plaque = elevated skin lesion, >1 cm in diameter. (see Fig. 1.3)

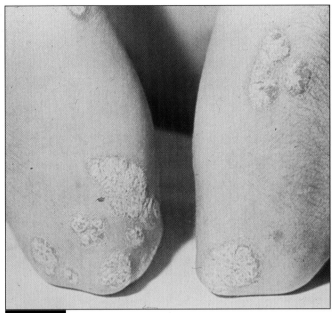

FIGURE 1.3

The silvery, scaly plaques of psoriasis tend to occur on the extensor surfaces, such as the elbows and knees. (courtesy of Dr. Douglas Smith)

4. Vesicle = small fluid-containing lesion, <0.5 cm in diameter. (see Fig. 1.4)

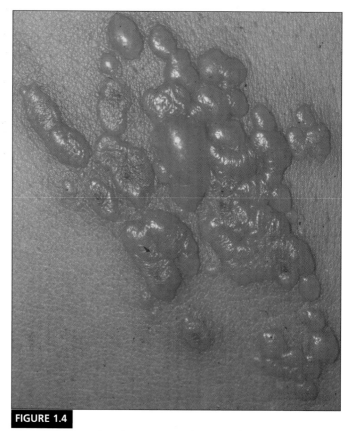

FIGURE 1.4

These vesicles are from herpes zoster. (courtesy of Dr. Steven Gammer)

5. Wheal = like a vesicle but occurs transiently as in urticaria (hives) (see Fig. 1.5)

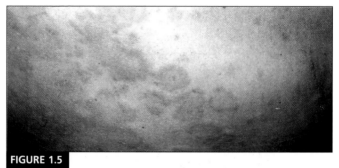

FIGURE 1.5

The ring-like wheals of urticaria. Reproduced with permission from Axford, J., Medicine. *Oxford, UK: Blackwell Science,1996.*

6. Bulla = large fluid-containing lesion, >0.5 cm in diameter. (see Fig. 1.6)

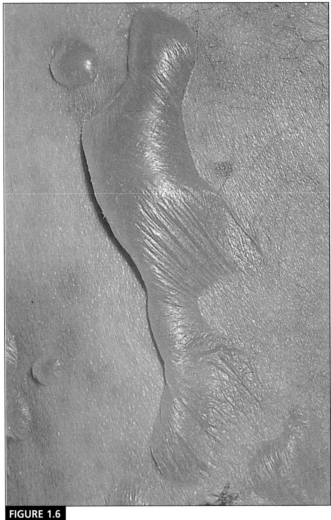

FIGURE 1.6

The large, tense bulla of bullous pemphigoid. Reproduced with permission from Axford, J., Medicine. Oxford, UK: Blackwell Science, 1996.

7. Lichenification = accentuated skin markings in thick epidermis, commonly due to scratching (see Fig. 1.7)

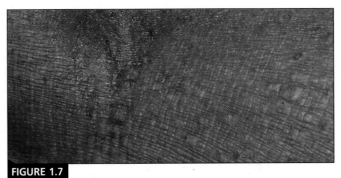

FIGURE 1.7

Chronic excoriation of eczema lead to lichenification in this patient. (courtesy of Dr. Steven Gammer)

8. Keloid = an irregular, raised lesion resulting from scar tissue hypertrophy, typically seen in dark-skinned individuals (see Fig. 1.8)

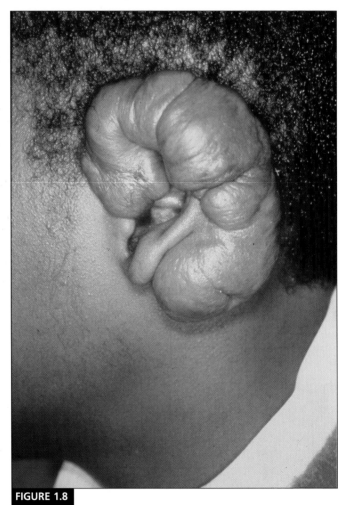

FIGURE 1.8

A traumatic injury to this dark-skinned patient's ear led to severe hypertrophic scar formation, otherwise known as keloid. (courtesy of Dr. Douglas Smith)

9. Petechiae = flat, pinhead, non-blanching, red-purple lesion caused by hemorrhage into the skin: seen in any cause of thrombocytopenia

10. Purpura = larger than petechiae

11. Cyst = closed epithelium-lined cavity or sac containing liquid or semi-solid material

12. Hyperkeratosis = ↑ thickness of stratum corneum (seen in chronic dermatitis and psoriasis) (see Fig. 1.9A)

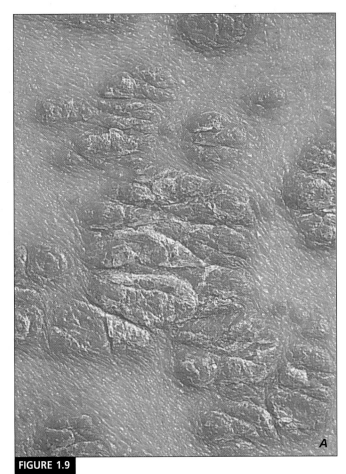

FIGURE 1.9

A) Hyperkeratosis is thickening of the stratum corneum.
Reproduced with permission from Axford, J., Medicine. Oxford, UK: Blackwell Science, 1996.

13. Parakeratosis = hyperkeratosis with retention of nuclei in stratum corneum and thinning of stratum granulosum (usually seen in psoriasis) (see Fig. 1.9B)

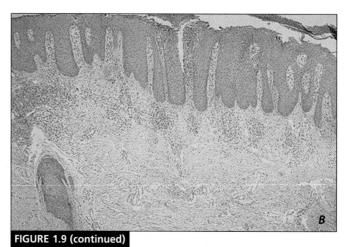

FIGURE 1.9 (continued)

B) Parakeratosis refers to retention of nuclei in the stratum corneum. Normally epidermal cells degrade and form pure collagen sheets in stratum corneum, but the rapid turnover of cell layers in psoriasis leads to desquamation prior to the degradation of epidermal cells. Reproduced with permission from Duncan, L., Dermatopathology CD-ROM. Malden, MA: Blackwell Science, 1998.

14. Acantholysis = loss of cohesion between epidermal cells (seen in pemphigus vulgaris)

15. Spongiosis = intercellular edema causing stretching and loss of desmosomal attachment, allowing formation of blisters within epidermis (seen in acute and subacute dermatitis) (see Fig. 1.10)

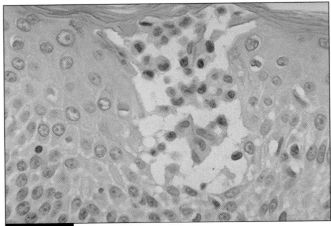

FIGURE 1.10

Edema contained within the epidermis is known as spongiosis. On histology this is seen as the presence of fluid collections between epidermal cells. Duncan, L., Dermatopathology CD-ROM. *Malden, MA: Blackwell Science,1998.*

16. Potency of Steroids

TABLE 1.1	Potency of Steroids	
POTENCY	**DRUG**	**USE FOR DISEASE ON. . .**
Low	1% hydrocortisone	face, genitals, skin folds (prevent atrophy/striae), also use in children for dz on body
Moderate	0.1% triamcinolone	body/extremities, or severe dz on face/genitals
High	Fluocinonide	thick skin (palms/soles), **do not use on face**
Very High	Diflorasone	thick skin, or if very severe on body
Carrier: lotion = low potency, cream = mid potency, ointment = high potency		

II. BACTERIAL INFECTIONS

A. Acne

1. Inflammation of pilosebaceous unit caused by secondary *Propionibacterium acnes* infection of blocked pore

2. Si/Sx = open comedones (blackheads) and closed comedones (whiteheads) on face, neck, chest, back, and buttocks, can become inflamed and pustular

3. Tx = topical antibiotics, Retin-A, benzoyl peroxide, systemic antibiotics, if acne is scarring consider Accutane

B. Impetigo

1. Superficial skin infection of epidermis

2. Si/Sx = honey crusted lesions or vesicles occurring most often in children around the nose and mouth, can be bullous or non-bullous (see Fig. 2.1)

3. Common organisms include *S. aureus* and *S. pyogenes*

4. Tx = first generation cephalosporin or nafcillin for 7–10 days

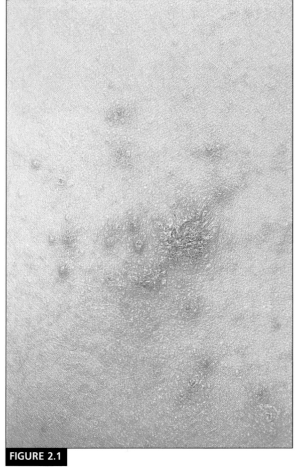

FIGURE 2.1

Impetigo presents with a golden or honey-colored crust over rup-tured vesicles or bullae. Reproduced with permission from Axford, J., Medicine. *Oxford, UK: Blackwell Science, 1996.*

C. Folliculitis

1. Si/Sx = erythematous pustules located directly over hair follicles

2. *S. aureus* most common, *Pseudomonas aeruginosa* causes "hot tub" folliculitis (organism lives in warm water), also fungi and viruses

3. Tx = local wound care, first generation cephalosporin only if severe

D. Subcutaneous Infections

1. Cellulitis

   a. Si/Sx = spreading subcutaneous infection with classic signs of inflammation: rubor (red), calor (hot), dolor (pain), and tumor (swelling)

   b. *Staphylococcus* and *Streptococcus* most common etiologies

   c. Tx = first generation cephalosporin or nafcillin

2. Erysipelas

   a. A type of cellulitis only with extension of infection to subcutaneous tissues, leading to edema localized beneath the infection

   b. Si/Sx = presents with bright red plaques with very sharp borders, classically affects the cheeks (unilateral or bilateral) (see Fig. 2.2), but can also affect other parts of the body

   c. Group A *Streptococcus* is the classic cause

   d. Tx = first generation cephalosporin

3. Abscess

   a. Local collection of pus, often with fever, ↑ white count

   b. Tx = incision and drainage (I&D) plus first generation cephalosporin

   c. Furuncle (boil) and Carbuncle

   d. Furuncle = pus collection in one hair follicle, often caused by *S. aureus*

   e. Carbuncle = pus collection involving many hair follicles

   f. Tx = I&D, add first generation cephalosporin or nafcillin if severe

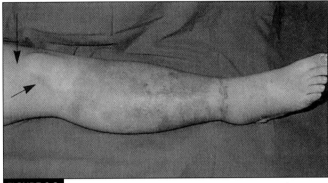

FIGURE 2.2

Erysipelas is a form of cellulitis characterized by local edema causing raised erythematous plaques instead of flat macules, with sharp borders. It is classically seen on the cheeks. Reproduced with permission from Axford, J., Medicine. Oxford, UK: Blackwell Science, 1996.

4. Paronychia

   a. Infxn of skin surrounding nail margin which can extend into surrounding skin and into tendons within hand

   b. Commonly caused by *S. aureus*, also *Candida*

   c. Tx = warm compress, I&D if area is purulent, add first generation cephalosporin if severe

5. Necrotizing fasciitis

   a. Infxn along fascial planes with severe pain, fever, ↑ white count, toxic-appearance to the pt, the classic clinical description is "pain out of proportion to the exam," meaning the pain is very severe in a spot where the inflammation doesn't look that bad

   c. Caused by *S. pyogenes* (Group A Strep) or *Clostridium perfringens*

   d. Tx = **immediate, extensive surgical débridement, add penicillin and clindamycin to help prevent further spread**

   e. Px = ↑↑↑ mortality unless débridement is rapid and extensive

E. Scarlet Fever

1. *Streptococcus pyogenes* (Group A *Strep* = GAS) causes a local infection (can be pharyngitis, etc.), and an immunologic reaction causes systemic illness

2. Si/Sx

   a. **"Sunburn with goose bumps"** rash, finely punctate, erythematous but blanches with pressure, initially on trunk, generalizes within hours

   b. Sandpaper rough skin, **strawberry tongue**, beefy red pharynx, circumoral pallor

   c. **Pastia's lines = lines of normal-colored skin in the creases of axillae and groin that stand out in contrast to the inflamed skin surrounding the creases**

   d. Eventual desquamation of hands and feet as rash resolves

   e. Systemic Sx include fever, chills, delirium, sore throat, cervical adenopathy, all of which appear at same time as rash

3. Complications include rheumatic fever and glomerulonephritis

4. Tx = penicillin

F. Hidradenitis Suppurativa

1. Si/Sx = plugged apocrine glands presenting as inflamed masses in groin/axilla, which can become secondarily infected

2. Tx = surgical débridement and antibiotics

G. Rose Spots

1. **Rose spots** = small pink papules in groups of 1–2 dozen on trunk, found in 30% of pts with typhoid fever (*Salmonella typhi*)

2. Typhoid Fever Si/Sx = high fever, myalgias, abdominal tenderness, splenomegaly, and **classic pulse–fever dissociation** = high fever with relative bradycardia

3. Tx = fluoroquinolone

H. Erythrasma

1. Can be seen in adult diabetics, caused by *Corynebacterium spp*

2. Si/Sx = irregular erythematous rash found along major skin folds (axilla, groin, fingers, toes, and breasts) (see Fig. 2.3)

3. Dx = Woods Lamp of skin → **coral red fluorescence, KOH Prep negative**

4. Tx = erythromycin

I. Mycobacterial Infection

1. Tuberculosis

   a. TB infection of the skin is called lupus vulgaris

   b. Si/Sx = erythematous macules or dusky-brown plaques, can present anywhere on the body

   c. Dx = biopsy is absolutely required to confirm the diagnosis, but it should be suspected in a patient with risks or signs and symptoms consistent with TB

   d. Tx = 4 drug TB therapy: isoniazid, rifampin, ethambutol, pyrazinamide

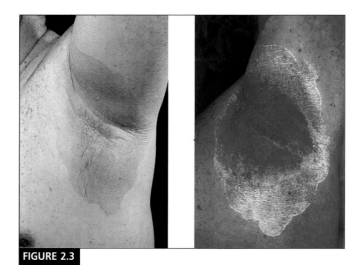

FIGURE 2.3

The shining of Woods Lamp ultraviolet light on the intertriginous rash leads to coral-red fluorescence. Reproduced with permission from Axford, J., Medicine. Oxford, UK: Blackwell Science, 1996.

2. Leprosy

   a. Several forms

      1) **Lepromatous is widely disseminated/poorly controlled infection in a host with minimal immune response**

      2) **Tuberculous occurs in hosts with good immune responses, leading to relative containment of bacterial infection**

      3) Intermediate forms also occur, not that these forms can convert into one another over time as the patient's immunity changes or as treatment is instituted

   b. Lepromatous Si/Sx = diffuse rash, can be large hypopigmented macules and/or nodules and plaques, **lesions are often focused in the cooler spots of the body, including the face, earlobes (leading to earlobe thickening)**

   c. Tuberculoid Si/Sx = hypopigmented macules that are also **anesthetic due to peripheral neuropathy,** and thickened peripheral nerves often palpable due to bacterial infestation of the nerves

   d. Tx = dapsone plus rifampin

III. COMMON BENIGN DISORDERS

A. Psoriasis

1. Si/Sx = pink plaques with silvery-white scaling **occurring on extensor surfaces, such as elbows and knees** (also scalp, lumbosacral, glans penis, intergluteal cleft) (see Fig. 1.3), **and fingernail pitting with onycholysis** (see Fig. 3.1), **can be associated with arthritis**

2. Classic finding = **Auspitz sign** → removal of overlying scale causes pinpoint bleeding due to thin epidermis above dermal papillae

3. Classic finding = **Koebner's phenomenon** → psoriatic lesions appear at sites of cutaneous physical trauma (skin scratching, rubbing, or wound)

4. Dx = clinical, biopsy is gold standard

5. Tx = topical steroids (first line), PUVA (second line) = **P**soralens + **UVA** light, methotrexate and cyclosporin (third line)

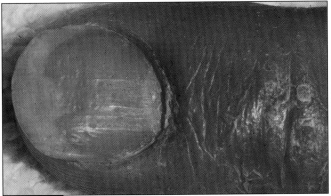

FIGURE 3.1

Involvement of the hands leads to pitting of the fingernails and onycholysis (lifting of the nail off the nailbed). (courtesy of Dr. Steven Gammer)

B. Eczema (Eczematous Dermatitis)

1. A family of superficial, intensely pruritic, erythematous skin lesions, including atopic dermatitis, contact dermatitis, seborrheic dermatitis

2. Atopic dermatitis

   a. Si/Sx = **an "itch that rashes,"** rash 2° to scratching chronic pruritus, **acutely get erythema and vesicles, subacutely get extensive weeping** of lesions as vesicles rupture **and** lots of **crusting**, chronically get **lichenification**

   b. Lesion distribution is commonly focused on the face in infancy, later in childhood can present on the flexor surfaces such as antecubital and popliteal fossa (see Fig. 3.2)

   c. Atopy = inherited predisposition to asthma, allergies, and dermatitis

   d. Dx is clinical

   e. Tx = avoid irritants or triggers, keep skin moist with lotions, use steroids and antihistamines for Sx relief of itching and inflammation

3. Contact dermatitis

   a. Si/Sx = linear pruritic rash at site of contact

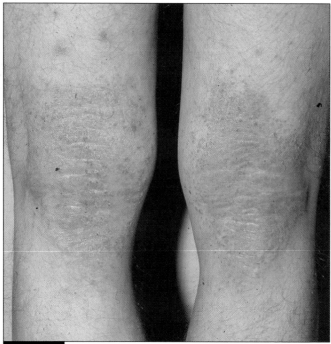

FIGURE 3.2

Chronic eczema presents with lichenification secondary to chronic excoriation. Note the distribution of these lesions in the popliteal fossae. (courtesy of Dr. Douglas Smith)

    b. Caused by Delayed Type Hypersensitivity reaction after exposure to poison ivy, poison oak, nickel, or chemicals

    c. Dx is clinical, history of exposure crucial

    d. Tx = as per atopic dermatitis

4. Seborrheic dermatitis

    a. Si/Sx = erythema, scaling, white flaking (dandruff) in areas of sebaceous glands (face, scalp, groin, axilla, and external ear), **most prominent throughout the face** (see Fig. 3.3)

    b. Called "Cradle Cap" in infants

    c. Dx = clinical and KOH prep to rule out fungal infection

    d. Tx = selenium shampoo on face and trunk, steroids for severe dz

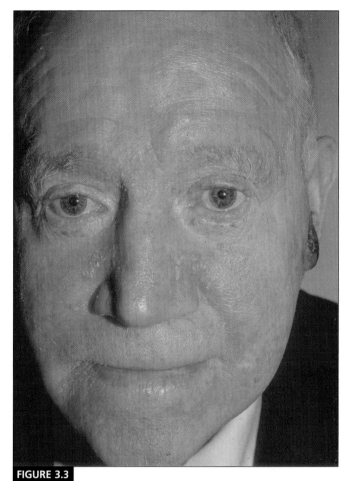

FIGURE 3.3

Classic seborrheic dermatitis affecting the face. (courtesy of Dr. Steven Gammer)

C. Urticaria (Hives)

1. Common disorder caused by mast cell degranulation and histamine release

2. Si/Sx = transient papular wheals, intensely pruritic, surrounded by erythema (see Figure 1.5), and **dermographism** (write word on the skin and it remains imprinted as erythematous wheals)

3. Most lesions are IgE-mediated (Type I Hypersensitivity) but exercise, certain chemicals in sensitive pts, and inhibitors of

prostaglandin synthesis (e.g., aspirin), can also cause IgE-independent reactions

4. Dx = skin testing or aspirin or exercise challenge
5. Tx = avoidance of triggers, antihistamines, steroids, epinephrine
6. Can cause respiratory emergency requiring intubation

D. Hypopigmentation

1. Vitiligo

   a. **Loss of melanocytes** in discrete areas of skin

   b. Si/Sx = sharply demarcated depigmented patches (see Fig. 3.4)

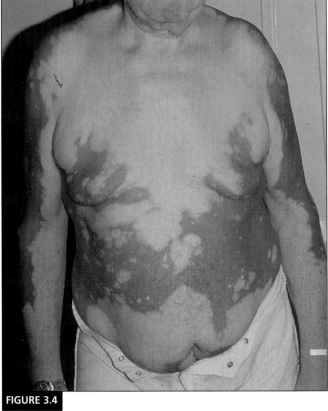

FIGURE 3.4

Extensive vitiligo. (courtesy of Dr. Steven Gammer)

   c. Occurs in all races but most apparent in darkly pigmented pts

   d. Chronic condition that may be autoimmune in nature

   e. Associated with thyroid dz in 30% of pts, especially women

   f. Tx = mini-grafting or total depigmentation

   g. Px = some patients remit over long term, others never do

2. Albinism

   a. **Melanocytes are present** but fail to produce pigment due to tyrosinase deficiency

   b. Si/Sx = white skin and eyelashes, nystagmus, iris translucency, ↓ visual acuity, decreased retinal pigment, and strabismus

   c. Tx = avoid sun exposure, sunscreens

   d. Px = the oculocutaneous form predisposes to skin cancer

3. Pityriasis alba

   a. Non-pathological areas of hypopigmentation on face or upper extremities

   b. Can be 2° to prior infection or inflammation, often regress over time

   c. Differentiated from Tinea versicolor by KOH prep

E. Hyperpigmentation

1. Freckle (ephelis) is caused by normal melanocyte number but ↑ melanin within basal keratinocytes, darkens with sun exposure

2. Lentigo is pigmented macules caused by melanocyte hyperplasia that, unlike freckles, do not darken with sun exposure

3. Nevo-cellular nevus

   a. Common mole, benign tumor derived from melanocytes

   b. Variations of nevi

      1) Blue nevus = black-blue nodule present at birth often mistaken for melanoma

      2) Spitz nevus = red-pink nodule, often seen in children, confused with hemangioma or melanoma

3) Dysplastic nevus = atypical, irregularly pigmented lesion with ↑ risk of transformation into malignant melanoma

   c. Dx = biopsy, Tx = full excision

4. Melasma (Chloasma)

   a. A mask-like hyperpigmentation on face seen in pregnancy

   b. Sunlight accentuates pigmentation which typically fades post-partum

   c. Tx = minimize facial exposure to sun, or hydroquinone cream (works for any hyperpigmentation)

5. Hemangioma

   a. Group of "birthmarks," capillary hemangiomas present at birth

   b. Port-wine stains (purple-red on face or neck)

     1) Can be associated with Sturge-Weber syndrome (see Phakomatoses below)

     2) Must screen for glaucoma and CNS dz (CT scan)

     3) Tx = laser therapy, will not regress spontaneously

   c. Strawberry hemangiomas (bright, raised, red lesions) are benign, most disappear on their own (see Fig. 3.5)

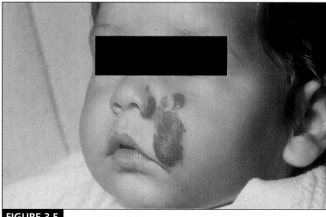

FIGURE 3.5

Cavernous hemangioma on the face. Reproduced with permission from Graham-Brown, R and Burns, T. Lecture Notes on Dermatology, *7th ed. Oxford, UK: Blackwell Science, 1996:154.*

    d. Cherry hemangiomas (benign, small, red papule) must Tx with laser therapy

6. Xanthoma

    a. Yellowish papules, often accumulations of foamy histiocytes (see Fig. 3.6)

    b. Can be idiopathic or associated with familial hyperlipidemia

    c. If seen on eyelids, they are called xanthelasma

    d. Tx = ↓ hyperlipidemia, surgically excise papules as needed

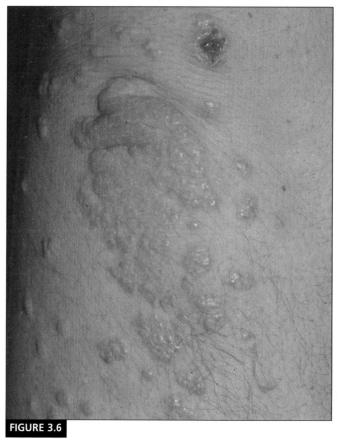

FIGURE 3.6

Multiple xanthoma (called eruptive xanthoma) in a patient with severe hypercholesterolemia. (courtesy of Dr. Steven Gammer)

7. Pityriasis rosea

    a. Erythematous maculopapular rash with scale apparent in center

    b. **Often preceded by a "herald patch" on trunk** (see inset to Fig. 3.7)

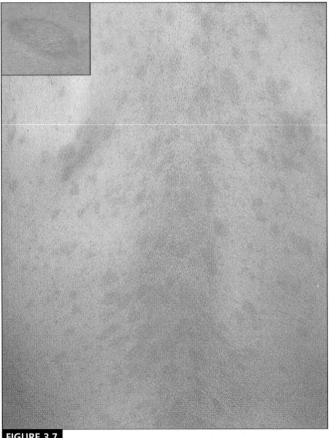

FIGURE 3.7

The herald patch (inset) of pityriasis rosea is typically found on the trunk and is much larger than the other papules (courtesy of Dr. Steven Gammer). Note the Christmas tree distribution of the lesions, following the skin lines in a concave shape up vertically close to the spine and horizontally along the sides. Reproduced with permission from Graham-Brown, R and Burns, T. Lecture Notes on Dermatology, 7th ed. *Oxford, UK: Blackwell Science, 1996:211.*

    c. **Appear on the trunk in a Christmas tree distribution,** following the skin lines concavely curving vertically up towards the spine and becoming horizontal towards the patient's sides (see Fig. 3.7)

    d. Tx = sunlight, otherwise spontaneously remits in 6-12 weeks

8. Erythema Nodosum

    a. Inflammation of subcutaneous fat (panniculitis) and adjacent vessels

    b. Characteristic lesions are **tender red nodules occurring on the lower legs,** and sometimes forearms (see Fig. 3.8)

    c. Usually resolves in 6–8 wks, Tx directed at underlying cause

    d. Common Causes

        1) Infections = *Mycoplasma, Chlamydia, Coccidioides immitis, Mycobacterium leprae* and in general, any granulomatous disease

        2) Drugs = sulfonamides and contraceptive pills

        3) Inflammatory Bowel Disease, sarcoidosis, rheumatic fever

        4) Pregnancy

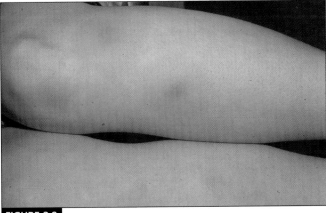

FIGURE 3.8

The red nodules of erythema nodosum classically occur on the shins. (courtesy of Dr. Steven Gammer)

9. Dermatomyositis

    a. An autoimmune disorder sometimes seen with polymyositis

    b. Presents with **heliotropic (reddish-purple) patches on eyelids** and erythematous scaly rash on hands

    c. Tx = high dose steroids

10. Seborrheic Keratosis

    a. **Black or brown benign plaques, appear to be stuck onto skin surface,** often occur extensively on the face (see Fig. 3.9A) and have a velvety/warty surface (see Fig. 3.9B)

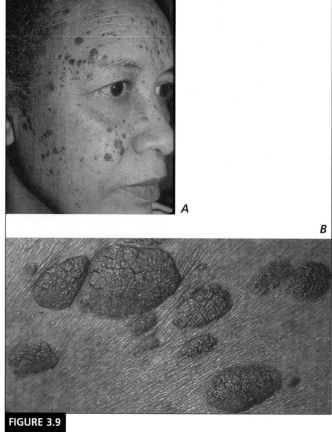

A

B

FIGURE 3.9

A) The black plaques of seborrheic keratosis appear to be "stuck-on." B) A close up of their velvety/warty surface. (both courtesy of Dr. Steven Gammer)

b. Commonly seen in elderly, and runs in families

c. Can be mistaken for melanoma

d. Tx = liquid nitrogen freezing, usually too many to treat

11. Acanthosis Nigricans

a. Fine, black velvety plaques on flexor surfaces and intertriginous areas (see Fig. 3.10)

b. Seen in obesity and endocrine disorders (e.g,. diabetes)

c. Can mark underlying malignancy (e.g., GI/GU, lymphoma)

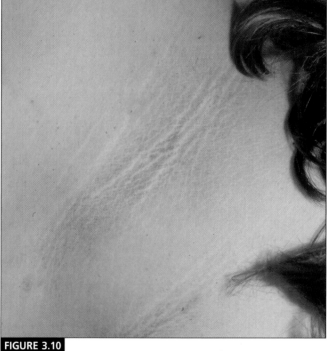

FIGURE 3.10

The fine, velvety plaque of acanthosis nigricans. (courtesy of Dr. Steven Gammer)

F. Verrucae (Warts)

1. Verruca Vulgaris = hand wart
2. Verruca Plana (Flat Wart) smaller than vulgaris, seen on hands and face
3. Human Papilloma Virus (HPV) types 1–4 cause skin and plantar warts
4. HPV 6 and 11 cause anorectal and genital warts (Condyloma Acuminatum)
5. HPV 16, 18, 31, 33, 35 cause cervical cancer
6. Condylomata lata are flat warts caused by *Treponema pallidum* (syphilis)

G. Sexually Transmitted Diseases

TABLE 3.1 **Sexually Transmitted Diseases**

DISEASE	CHARACTERISTICS	TX
Chancroid (*Hemophilus ducreyi*)	• Si/Sx = genital ulcer, looks like syphilitic chancre, but **unlike chancre, chancroid is very painful** • Dx = clinical or biopsy	• 3rd generation cephalosporin or macrolide
Gonorrhea (*Neisseria gonorrhea*)	• Si/Sx = gonococcemia results in **scattered pustules, frequently on the palms and soles** • Dx = gram stain of urethral discharge, blood cultures, or biopsy of skin lesion	• 3rd generation cephalosporin
Herpes Simplex Virus (HSV)	• Si/Sx = **painful vesicles and ulcers,** 1° infxn →malaise, fever, inguinal adenopathy in 40% of patients • Dx confirmed with direct fluorescent antigen (DFA) staining, Tzanck prep, serology, HSV PCR, or culture	• Tx = acyclovir, famciclovir, or valacyclovir

TABLE 3.1	Sexually Transmitted Diseases (continued)	
DISEASE	**CHARACTERISTICS**	**TX**
HIV	• Si/Sx = seroconversion can present with diffuse erythematous maculopapular rash • 2° infections include thrush, *Candida* intertriginous infections, tinea pedis (foot infections), onychomycosis, regular cellulitis, other sexually transmitted diseases • **Psoriasis, seborrheic dermatitis, and molluscum contagiosum are much more severe in AIDS pts** • **AIDS pts commonly get a severe folliculitis called eosinophilic folliculitis** • Kaposi' s sarcoma is common and extensive in AIDS pts • All skin cancers are more common in AIDS pts	• Highly Active Anti-Retroviral Therapy (HAART) and Tx the skin disease as usual
Human Papillomavirus (HPV)	• Spread by direct skin-to-skin contact • Si/Sx = condyloma acuminata (genital warts) = soft, fleshy growths on vagina, cervix, perineum, and anus • Dx = clinical, confirmed with biopsy	• Topical podophyllin or trichloracetic acid, if refractory → cryosurgery or excision
Lympho-granuloma Venereum (*Chlamydia trachomatis*)	• Si/Sx = extensive inguinal adenopathy that leads to the classic **"groove sign,"** which is a groove of skin folded underneath massive lymphadenopathy on either side of the inguinal ligament	• Doxycycline or azithromycin
Syphilis (*Treponema pallidum*)	• Si/Sx 1° dz = **chancre, a painless ulcer** • 2° dz = 4 to 8 weeks later → fever, lymphadenopathy, **maculopapular rash affecting palms and soles, condyloma lata in intertriginous area**s • 3° dz = years later → gummas • Dx = VDRL/RPR for screening, FTA-ABS to confirm	• Benzathine penicillin G

IV. CANCER

TABLE 4.1	Skin Cancers		
DISEASE	**SI/SX**	**TX**	**PX**
Basal Cell Carcinoma	• Most common skin cancer • Si/Sx = classic **"Rodent ulcer"** on face, **with pearly translucent borders and fine telangiectasias** (see Fig. 4.1)	excision	excellent—almost never metastasize
Squamous Cell Carcinoma	• Common in elderly • Si/Sx = erythematous nodules on sun exposed areas that eventually ulcerate and crust (see Fig. 4.2) • **Frequently preceded by Actinic Keratosis = rough epidermal lesions on sun exposed areas**	excision, radiation	metastasize more then basal cell but not as much as melanoma
Malignant Melanoma	• Seen in lightly pigmented individuals with ↑ sun exposure –diagnose with **ABCDEs** • **A**symmetry = malignant, benign = symmetrical • **B**order = irregular, benign = smooth borders • **C**olor = multicolored, benign = one color • **D**iameter >6mm, benign = <6 mm • **E**levation = raised above skin, benign = flat • **E**nlargement = growing, benign = not growing (see Fig. 4.3)	excision, chemo if mets likely	high rate of metastasis → **#1 skin cancer killer, risk of mets ↑ with depth of invasion on biopsy**
Kaposi' s Sarcoma	• Caused by Human Herpes Virus 8 • Si/Sx = red/purple plaques or nodules on skin and mucosa, frequently affects lungs and GI viscera, **almost exclusively seen in AIDS patients (see Fig. 4.4)**	HIV drugs, chemo	benign unless damages internal organs
Cutaneous T-Cell Lymphoma	• Also known as **"Mycosis Fungoides"** • Si/Sx = **pink, scaly patches or nodules that may ulcerate (see Fig. 4.5) or develop into systemic erythroderma** (total body erythematous and pruritic rash)	PUVA, topical chemo, radiation	7–10 yr life expectancy without Tx

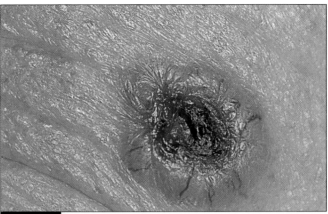

FIGURE 4.1

The rodent ulcer of basal cell carcinoma. Note the telangietasias at the borders. Reproduced with permission from Axford, J., Medicine. Oxford, UK: Blackwell Science,1996.

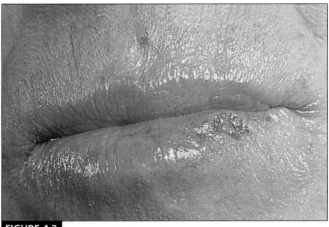

FIGURE 4.2

Squamous cell carcinoma of the lip (early ulcer). Reproduced with permission from Axford, J., Medicine. Oxford, UK: Blackwell Science,1996.

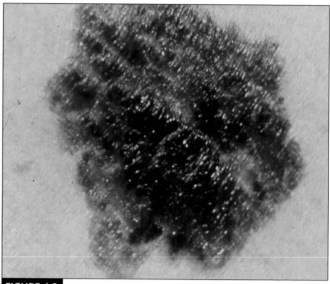

FIGURE 4.3

A melanoma with the ABCDEs. The lesion is Asymmetric, with irregular Borders, is multiColored, has a large Diameter, and is Elevated (plaque not macule). It was also Enlarging. (courtesy of Dr. Douglas Smith)

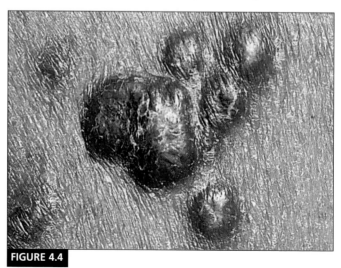

FIGURE 4.4

The red/purple nodules of Kaposi's sarcoma. Reproduced with permission from Axford, J., Medicine. Oxford, UK: Blackwell Science, 1996.

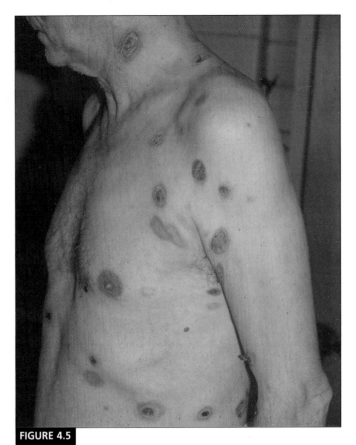

FIGURE 4.5

The pink patches of Mycosis Fungoides can ulcerate. (courtesy of Dr. Steven Gammer)

V. NEUROCUTANEOUS SYNDROMES (PHAKOMATOSES)

1. Tx is supportive depending upon individual signs and symptoms

TABLE 5.1 Phakomatoses	
DISEASE*	**CHARACTERISTICS**
Tuberous Sclerosis	**Ash leaf patches** (hypopigmented macules) (see **Fig. 5.1A**), **Shagreen spots** (leathery cutaneous thickening), **adenoma sebaceum** of the face (**see Fig. 5.1B**), **seizures, mental retardation**
Neurofibromatosis (NF)	**Café-au-lait spots, neurofibromas** (**see Fig. 5.2**), meningiomas, acoustic neuromas, kyphoscoliosis— NF 2 causes bilaterial acoustic neuromas
Sturge-Weber Syndrome	**Port-wine hemangioma of face** in CN V distribution, mental retardation, seizures
von Hippel-Lindau Syndrome	Multiple hemangiomas in various organs, ↑ frequency of renal cell CA and polycythemia (↑ erythropoietin secretion)
*All are autosomal dominant except Sturge-Weber, which has no genetic pattern.	

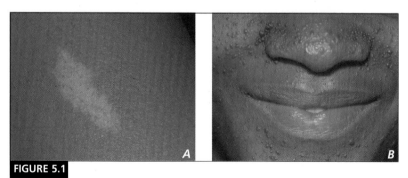

FIGURE 5.1

The ash leaf patch (A) and adenoma sebaceum (B) characteristic of tuberous sclerosis. (both courtesy of Dr. Steven Gammer)

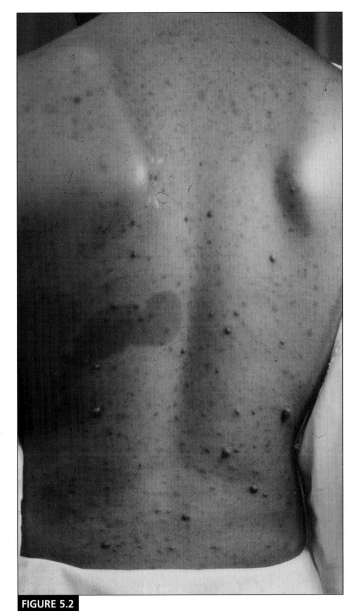

FIGURE 5.2

Several neurofibromas and a large café-au-lait spot. (courtesy of Dr. Steven Gammer)

VI. BLISTERING DISORDERS

A. Pemphigus Vulgaris (PG)

1. PG is a rare autoimmune disorder, **affecting 20–40 yo**

2. Si/Sx = **flaccid epidermal bullae that easily slough off leaving large denuded areas of skin** (see Fig. 6.1A), **also present is Nikolsky's Sign**in that the skin sloughs off with only minor pressure (see Fig. 6.1B), ↑ risk of 2° infxn

3. DDx = Bullous Pemphigoid

4. Dx = skin biopsy → **immunofluorescence surrounding epidermal cells** showing "tombstone fluorescent pattern"

5. Tx = high dose oral steroids, antibiotics for infection

6. Px = **often fatal if not treated**

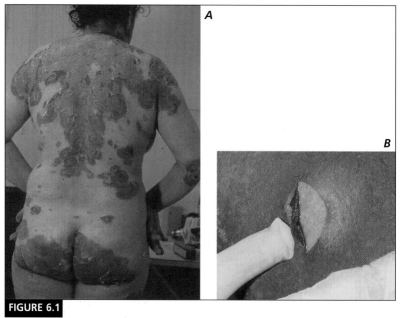

FIGURE 6.1

A) The flaccid bullae of pemphigus vulgaris slough easily, leaving inflamed, denuded areas of skin. B) Nikolsky's sign is present due to the weak attachments of the bullae to the underlying epidermis. (both courtesy of Dr. Steven Gammer)

B. Bullous Pemphigoid (BP)

1. Common autoimmune disease affecting **mostly the elderly**

2. Resembles PG but much less severe clinically

3. Si/Sx = **hard, tense bullae** that do not rupture easily and usually heal without scarring if uninfected (see Figure 1.6 and Figure 6.2)

4. Dx = Skin biopsy → immunofluorescence as a **linear band along the basement membrane, with** ↑ **eosinophils** in dermis

5. Tx = oral steroids

6. Px = much better then PG

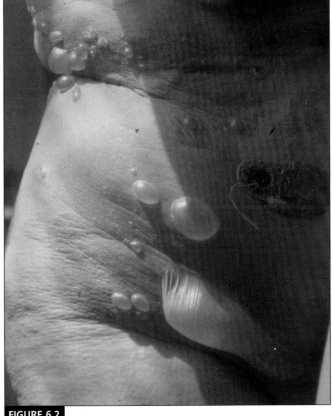

FIGURE 6.2

Multiple tense bullae of bullous pemphigoid. (courtesy of Dr. Steven Gammer)

C. Erythema Multiforme

1. A hypersensitivity reaction to drugs, infections, or systemic disorders, such as malignancy or collagen vascular disease

2. Si/Sx = **diffuse, erythematous target-like lesions** (see Fig. 6.3A) in many shapes (hence name Multiforme), often accompanying a herpes eruption

3. **Stevens-Johnson Syndrome = a severe febrile form (sometimes fatal) → hemorrhagic crusting also affects lips and oral mucosa** (see Fig. 6.3B)

4. Dx = clinical, hx of herpes infection or drug exposure

5. Tx = stop offending drug, prevent eruption of herpes with acyclovir

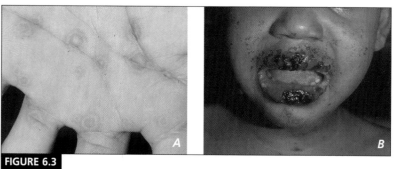

FIGURE 6.3

A) The target-like lesions of erythema multiforme. B) Stevens-Johnson syndrome is a more severe presentation of erythema multiforme, in which mucosal surfaces are involved as well. (both courtesy of Dr. Steven Gammer)

D. Cutaneous Porphyria Tarda

1. Autosomal dominant defect in heme synthesis (50% ↓ in uroporphyrinogen decarboxylase activity in RBC and liver)

2. Si/Sx = blisters on sun exposed areas of face and hands, ↑ hair on temples and cheeks, **no abdominal pain** (differentiates from other porphyrias)

3. Dx = Woods Lamp of urine → **urine fluoresces with distinctive orange-pink color due to** ↑ **levels of uroporphyrins**

4. Tx = sunscreen, phlebotomy, chloroquine, no alcohol

5. Px = remitting/relapsing, exacerbations due to viral hepatitis, hepatoma, alcohol abuse, estrogen, sunlight

VII. VECTOR-BORNE DISEASES

A. Bacillary Angiomatosis (Peliosis Hepatis)

1. Si/Sx = weight loss, abdominal pain, **rash = red or purple vascular lesions**, from papule to hemangioma-sized, located anywhere on skin and disseminated to any organ

2. DDx = Kaposi sarcoma, cherry hemangioma

3. **Almost always seen in HIV⊕ patients or homeless population**

4. Caused by *Bartonella spp.*, leading to dysregulated angiogenesis

5. **Cat-scratch disease caused by *B. henselae* transmitted by kitten scratches, Trench Fever caused by *B. quintana* spread by lice**

6. Dx = histopathology with silver stain, visualization of organisms in lesion, blood culture and PCR can also be done

7. Tx = erythromycin

8. Px = excellent with Tx, some pts require lifelong suppressive Tx

B. Lyme Disease

1. Si/Sx = fever, chills, headaches, lethargy, photophobia, meningitis, myocarditis, arthralgia, and myalgias

2. **Classic rash = erythema chronicum migrans → erythematous annular plaques with a red migrating border and central clearing and induration**

3. Dx = PCR for *Borrelia burgdorferi* DNA, or skin biopsy of migrating edge looking for causative spirochete

4. Tx = spray skin and clothes with DEET or permethrin, wear long pants in woods to prevent tick bite (*Ixodes dammini* and *Ixodes pacificus*)

5. Once infected → high dose penicillin or ceftriaxone for 2–4 wks

C. Rocky Mountain Spotted Fever

1. Si/Sx = acute onset fever, headache, myalgias, classic rash

2. Rash = **erythematous maculopapular, starting on wrists and ankles then moving towards palms, soles, and trunk**

3. Rash may lead to cutaneous necrosis due to DIC-induced occlusion of small cutaneous vessels with thrombi

4. Dx = by Hx (exposure to outdoors or tick bite, *Dermacentor spp.*), serologies for *Rickettsia rickettsii*, skin biopsy

5. Doxycycline or chloramphenicol

VIII. PARASITIC INFECTIONS

A. Scabies

1, Si/Sx = **erythematous, markedly pruritic papules and burrows located intertriginous areas** (e.g., finger and toe webs, groin) (see Fig. 8.1), lesions contagious

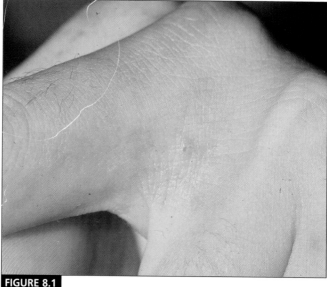

FIGURE 8.1

A papule located in the finger web is classic for scabies. (courtesy of Dr. Steven Gammer)

2. Dx = microscopic identification of *Sarcoptes scabiei* mite in skin scrapings

3. Tx = Pt and all close contacts apply Permethrin 5% cream to entire body for 8–10 hrs then repeat in one wk, wash all bedding in hot water the same day

4. Lindane cream is less effective, associated with adverse effects in kids

5. Symptomatic relief of hypersensitivity reaction to dead mites may be treated with antihistamines and topical steroids

B. Pediculosis Capitis (Head Louse)

1. Si/Sx = can be asymptomatic, or pruritus and erythema of scalp may be noted, common in school-aged children

2. Dx = microscope exam of hair shaft (see Fig. 8.2), nits may fluoresce with Woods Lamp

3. Permethrin shampoo or gel to scalp, may need to repeat

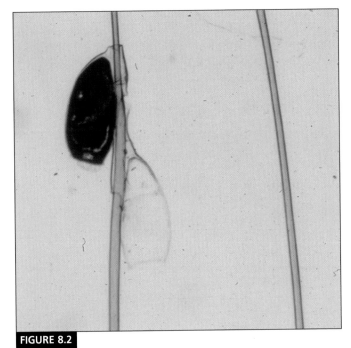

FIGURE 8.2

A louse and an empty casing attached to hair shaft. (courtesy of Dr. Steven Gammer)

C. Pediculosis Pubis "Crabs"

1. Si/Sx = very **pruritic papules in pubic area**, axilla, periumbilically in males, along eyelashes, eyebrows, and buttocks

2. Dx = microscopic identification of lice, rule out other STDs

3. Tx = apply Permethrin 5% shampoo for 10 minutes then repeat in one week

D. Cutaneous Larva Migrans (Creeping Eruption)

1. Si/Sx = erythematous, pruritic, **serpiginous thread-like lesion** marking burrow of migrating nematode larvae, often on back, hands, feet, buttocks (see Fig. 8.3)

2. Organism = hookworms: *Ancylostoma*, *Necator*, and *Strongyloides*

3. Dx = Hx of unprotected skin laying in moist soil or sand, Tx of lesion

4. Tx = ivermectin orally or thiabendazole topically

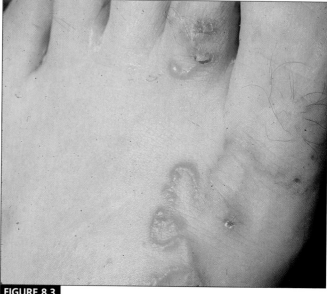

FIGURE 8.3

The serpiginous, subcutaneous parasite of cutaneous larva migrans. (courtesy of Dr. Steven Gammer)

IX. FUNGAL CUTANEOUS DISORDERS

TABLE 9.1	Fungal Infections		
DISEASE	**SI/SX**	**DX**	**TX**
Tinea	• Erythematous, pruritic, scaly, well-demarcated plaques (see Fig. 9.1) • Black dots may be seen on scalp of patients with Tinea capitis	Clinical or KOH prep	Topical antifungal (oral needed for Tinea capitis)
Onycho-mycosis	• Finger or toenails appear thickened, yellow, degenerating	Clinical or KOH prep	PO itraconazole or griseofulvin
Tinea versicolor	• Caused by *Pityrosporum ovale* • Multiple macules with sharp margins on face and trunk, **hyperpigmented in light-skinned individuals and hyperpigmented in dark-skinned individuals** (see Fig. 9.2)	KOH prep →yeast and hyphae with classic **spaghetti and meatball** appearance	Selenium sulfide shampoo daily to affected areas for seven days
Candida	• Erythematous scaling plaques, often in intertriginous areas (groin, breast, buttocks, web of hands), **always have "satellite lesions" located beyond border of main infection (see Fig. 9.3)** • Oral thrush →cottage-cheese-like white plaques on mucosal surface • Can extend to esophagus and cause dysphagia and odynophagia	KOH prep →Budding yeast and pseudo-hyphae	Topical Nystatin or oral fluconazole

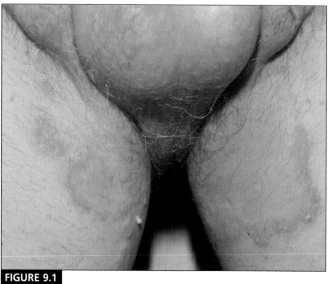

FIGURE 9.1

Tinea cruris (tinea in the groin) is shown here. It has well demarcated, scaly plaques and has no satellite lesions. (courtesy of Dr. Steven Gammer)

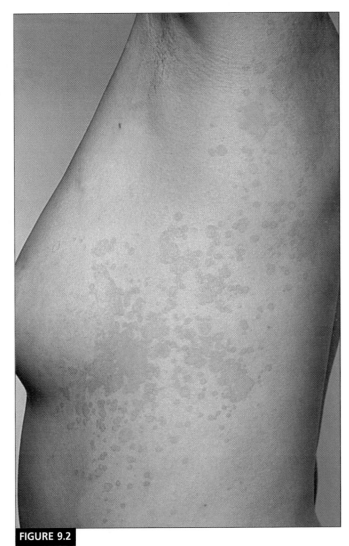

FIGURE 9.2

Pityriasis versicolor Petaloid, scaly macules. Reproduced with permission from Axford, J., Medicine. Oxford, UK: Blackwell Science,1996.

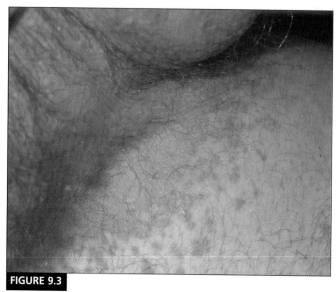

FIGURE 9.3

An erythematous intertriginous infection is usually Candida *if there are "satellite lesions" beyond the edges of the main infection. (courtesy of Dr. Steven Gammer)*

X. VIRAL EXANTHEMS

TABLE 10.1	Viral Exanthems

DISEASE	CHARACTERISTICS
Measles (Rubeola)	• Caused by a **paramyxovirus** • Si/Sx = erythematous maculopapular rash, erupts about five days after onset of prodromal symptoms, **pathognomonic Koplik spots are white spots on an erythematous base on the buccal mucosa,** but these disappear when the rash begins and so are usually not found on presentation • Measles rash begins on the head and spreads downward, lasting 4–5 days and resolving from the head downward • **Dx = the 3 Cs: cough, coryza, conjunctivitis ⊕fever**
Molluscum Contagiosum	• Caused by a poxvirus • Si/Sx = pearly papules with central umbilication **(see Fig. 1.2)**, in AIDS pts the virus disseminates rapidly, leading to multiple patches of papules
Rubella (German Measles)	• Caused by a **togavirus** • **Presents with suboccipital lymphadenopathy** (one of the very few diseases to do this) and maculopapular rash that begins on face and then generalizes, lasts 5 days
Hand, Foot, and Mouth Disease	• Caused by **Coxsackie A** virus • Vesicular rash on hands and feet with ulcerations in the mouth, clearing in about a week **(see Fig. 10.1)**
Roseola infantum (exanthem subitum)	• Caused by **Herpes Virus 6** • Often begins with **abrupt high fever persisting for 1–5 days even though child has no physical signs to account for fever and does not feel malaised,** rash doesn't appear until the fever goes away and often resolves within 24 hours
Erythema Infectiosum (Fifth Disease)	• Caused by **Parvovirus B-19** • **Classic finding is "Slapped Cheeks,"** erythema of the cheeks • Subsequently an erythematous maculopapular rash involves the arms and spreads to trunk and legs forming a reticular pattern • This disease may be dangerous in Sickle Cell pts (and other anemias) due to Parvovirus B-19's tendency to cause aplastic crises in such patients

TABLE 10.1	Viral Exanthems (continued)
DISEASE	**CHARACTERISTICS**
Varicella (Chicken Pox)	• Caused by the **Varicella-Zoster Virus**, a type of herpes virus • Highly contagious, pruritic "tear drop" vesicles that break and crust over, beginning on face or trunk (centripetal) and spreading towards extremities • New lesions appear for 3–5 days and typically take three days to crust over, so rash persists for about one week • **Lesions are contagious until they crust over** • Zoster (Shingles) represents a reactivation of an old varicella infection • Painful skin eruptions are seen along the distribution of dermatomes that correspond to the affected dorsal root ganglia (**see Fig. 10.2**)

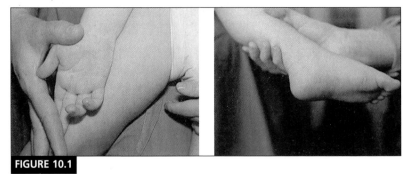

FIGURE 10.1

The typical blisters of hand, foot, and mouth disease. Reproduced with permission from Bannister et al., Infectious Disease. *Oxford, UK: Blackwell Science,1996.*

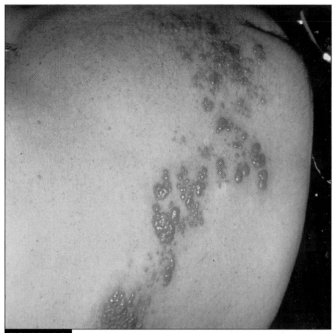

FIGURE 10.2

The dermatomal distribution to these vesicles on an erythematous base is pathognomonic for herpes zoster. (courtesy of Dr. Steven Gammer)

REVIEW QUESTIONS

1. Match the following terms with their appropriate definitions:

   a. Macule   1. small, fluid-filled lesion

   b. Bulla   2. accentuated skin markings

   c. Vesicle   3. large, fluid-filled lesion

   d. Hyperkeratosis   4. thickened stratum corneum

   e. Lichenification   5. flat, colored lesion

2. A classic description of necrotizing fasciitis is:

   a. The flesh eating virus

   b. Diffuse sloughing of skin

   c. Gas formation

   d. Pain out of proportion to the exam

   e. Ulceration of the overlying skin

3. All of the following are physical findings of scarlet fever **except:**

   a. Strawberry tongue

   b. Pastia's lines

   c. "Sunburn with goose bumps"

   d. Desquamation

   e. Follicular erythema

4. Which of the following causes of intertriginous infection fluoresces coral-red under Wood's Lamp?

   a. *Corynebacterium spp.*

   b. *Candida albicans*

   c. Tinea cruris

   d. Tinea versicolor

   e. *Malassezia furfur*

5. Match the following diseases with their classic finding or descriptor:

   a. Psoriasis   1. facial erythema

   b. Eczema   2. transient wheals

   c. Seborrheic dermatitis   3. silvery plaques on elbows

   d. Urticaria   4. "an itch that rashes"

6. Match the following diseases with their classic physical findings:

   a. Dermatomyositis   1. Rose spots

   b. Typhoid fever   2. warty, "stuck-on" lesions

   c. Erythema nodosum   3. painful, red nodules on shins

   d. Seborrheic keratosis   4. heliotropic rash around eyes

   e. Acanthosis nigricans   5. velvety, intertriginous plaques

7. Match the following sexually transmitted diseases with their characteristic physical findings:

   a. Syphilis   1. verrucae

   b. Herpes   2. groove sign

   c. Gonorrhea   3. painful ulcer on penis

   d. Chancroid   4. maculopapular lesions on palms and soles

   e. HPV   5. painful vesicles

   f. Chlamydia   6. folliculitis

   g. HIV   7. urethral discharge

8. Which of the following statements regarding skin cancers are **not** true?

   a. Basal cell carcinoma and squamous cell carcinoma rarely metastasize

   b. Melanoma has a poor prognosis due to its high incidence of metastases

   c. The most important prognostic marker of melanoma metastasis is the depth of malignant invasion on biopsy, **not** the diameter of the lesion on the skin surface

   d. Kaposi's sarcoma always occurs in AIDS patients

   e. Cutaneous T cell Lymphoma is also known as Mycosis Fungoides

9. Match the following viral infections with their classic signs and symptoms:

   a. Measles   1. slapped cheeks

   b. Molluscum contagiosum   2. suboccipital
                                    lymphadenopathy

   c. Rubella   3. cough, coryza,
                                    conjunctivitis

   d. Roseola infantum   4. pearly papules with umbil-
                                    ication

   e. Erythema infectiosum   5. rash appears after fever
                                    resolves

10. Which of the following statements regarding blistering disorders is **not** true?

    a. The bullae of pemphigus vulgaris slough easily

    b. Bullous pemphigoid affects older patients than pemphigus vulgaris, and thus has a worse prognosis

    c. Erythema multiforme presents with bulls-eye or target lesions

    d. Cutaneous porphyria tarda does **not** present with abdominal pain

ANSWERS

1. **a-5, b-3, c-1, d-4, e-2**. See terminology section for descriptions.

2. **d)** Necrotizing fasciitis is a severe infection of fascial plains. Gas formation is not a common feature, nor is sloughing of overlying skin. The appearance of necrotizing fasciitis is erythema with vague borders, and severe pain on palpation of the area, despite the relatively mild appearance.

3. **e)** Follicular erythema refers to folliculitis. The other findings are seen in scarlet fever.

4. **a)** Erythrasma is an intertriginous infection caused by a *Corynebacterium*, which fluoresces coral-red under Wood's Lamp. It is otherwise difficult to distinguish this infection from tinea cruris or *Candida*. Tinea versicolor does not cause intertriginous infections. *Malassezia furfur* is a species name of the organism that causes Tinea versicolor.

5. **a-3, b-4, c-1, d-2**.

6. **a-4, b-1, c-3, d-2, e-5**.

7. **a-4** (1 also acceptable), **b-5, c-7, d-3, e-1, f-2, g-6**. One of the favorite things to do on the Boards is to present a case of a sexually promiscious person with a new onset of a painful ulcer on the tip of the vagina or penis. The first thing that leaps to mind is syphilis. Don't be fooled! The chancre lesion of syphilis is **painless**, not painful! Chancroid causes a lesion that can appear identical to a chancre but is painful. Syphilis can also cause verrucae, called condyloma lata, which are typically found in the anus or vagina. Gonorrhea causes urethral discharge. Disseminated gonococcemia can cause pustular lesions on the palms and soles, but not maculopapular lesions, which are a classic description of the rash of secondary syphilis. HIV causes eosinophilic folliculitis, and HPV causes condyloma acuminata, while Herpes causes painful vesicles. Lymphogranuloma venereum, caused by *Chlamydia*, presents with massive inguinal adenopathy, causing the groove sign, which is a groove formed along the line of the inguinal ligament by the adenopathy on either side of the ligament.

8. **d)** Although Kaposi's sarcoma is most commonly seen in AIDS patients, a distinct variety occurs in older men of Mediterranean extraction. Remember, by far the most important prognostic feature of melanoma is its depth of invasion in the skin. The diameter of the lesion on the surface is a less reliable prognostic indicator.

9 a-3, b-4, c-2, d-5, e-1.

10. **b)** Bullous pemphigoid does occur in older patients than pemphigus vulgaris, but the prognosis of bullous pemphigoid is much better than pemphigus vulgaris because the bullae of bullous pemphigoid tend not to rupture. Because the bullae of pemphigus rupture so easily, they leave behind denuded skin, allowing dehydration and infection to set in.

INDEX

Note: Page numbers followed by *t* refer to tables.

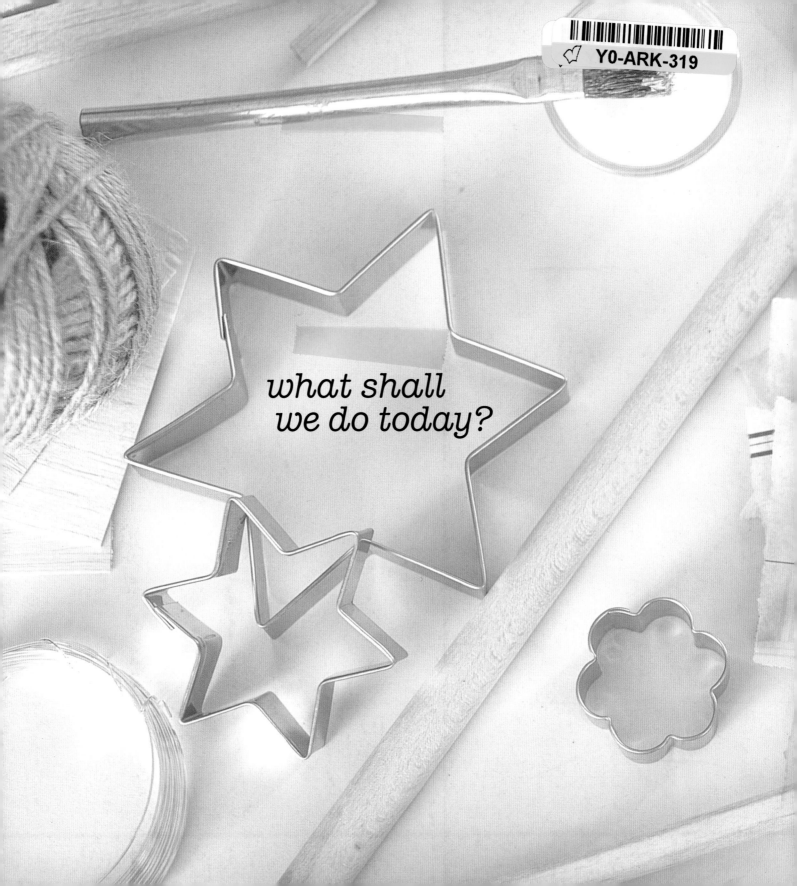

what shall
we do today?

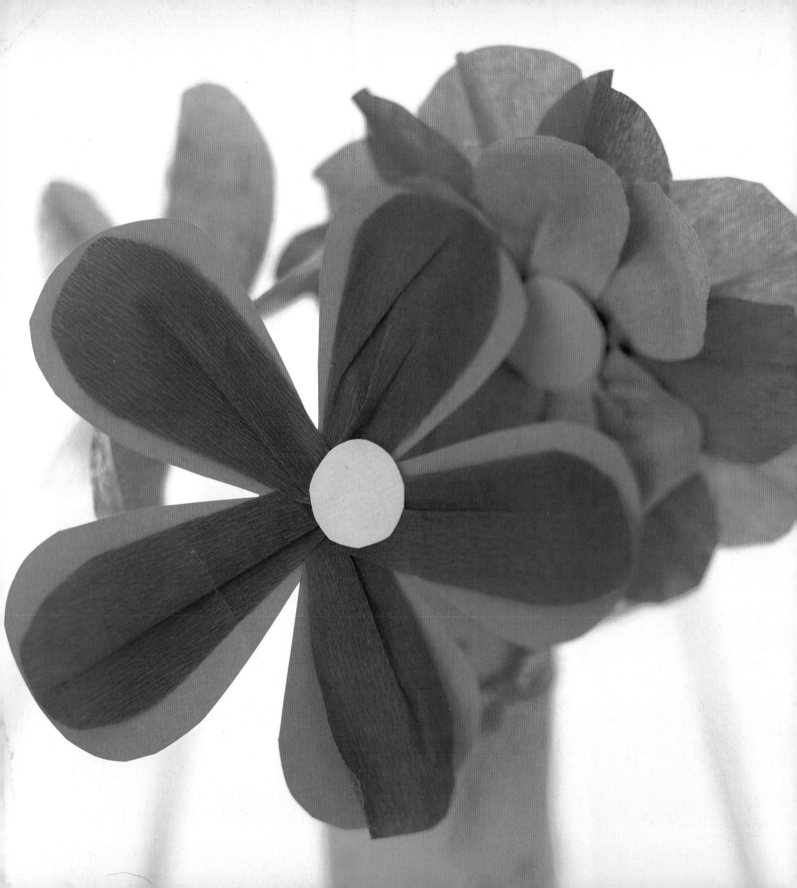

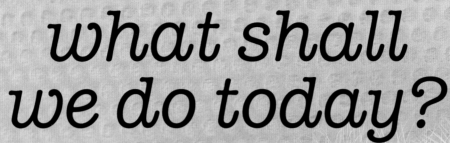

what shall we do today?

with projects by
Catherine Woram

RYLAND
PETERS
& SMALL

LONDON NEW YORK

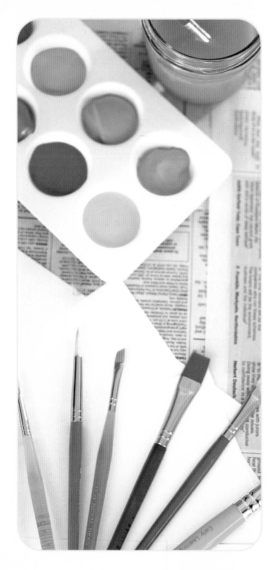

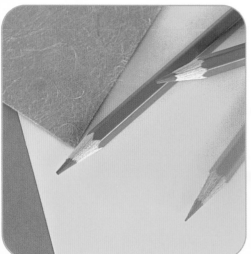

Designer Iona Hoyle
Commissioning editor Annabel Morgan
Picture research Emily Westlake
Production Hazel Kirkman
Art director Leslie Harrington
Publishing director Alison Starling

Stylist Catherine Woram

First published in the United States in 2009
by Ryland Peters and Small, Inc
519 Broadway, Fifth Floor
New York, NY 10012
www.rylandpeters.com

10 9 8 7 6 5 4

Text, design and photographs
© Ryland Peters & Small 2009, except the recipes
on pages 26–27 and 126–127, which are both
copyright © Linda Collister 2009

All the projects in this book are by Catherine
Woram, except the recipes on pages 26–27 and
126–127, which are both by Linda Collister.
The projects in this book have been published
previously by Ryland Peters & Small in *Baking with
Kids*, *Christmas Crafting with Kids*, *Cooking with
Kids*, *Crafting with Kids*, and *Gardening with Kids*.

ISBN: 978-1-84597-887-7

Library of Congress Cataloging-in-Publication
Data

Woram, Catherine.
  What shall we do today? / with projects by
Catherine Woram.
    p. cm.
  Includes index.
  ISBN 978-1-84597-887-7
  1. Handicraft--Juvenile literature. I. Title.
  TT160.W68 2009
  745.5--dc22
                                          2009015913

Printed and bound in China

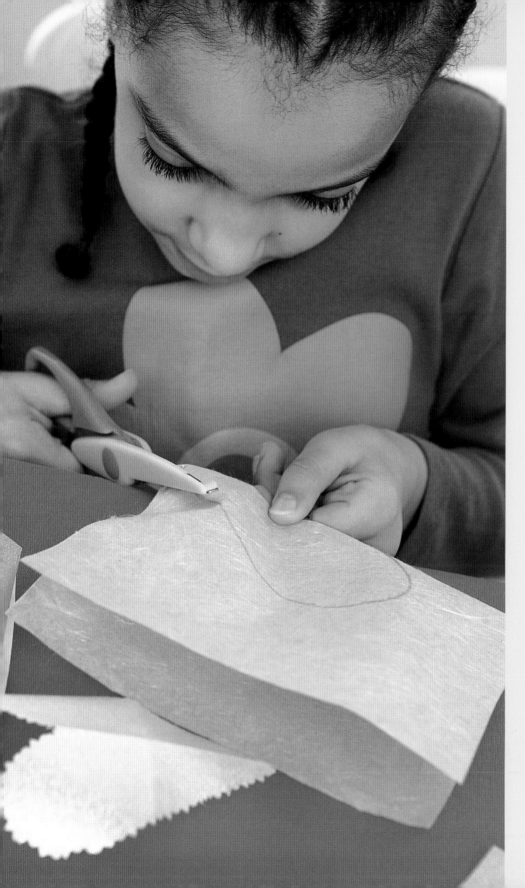

contents

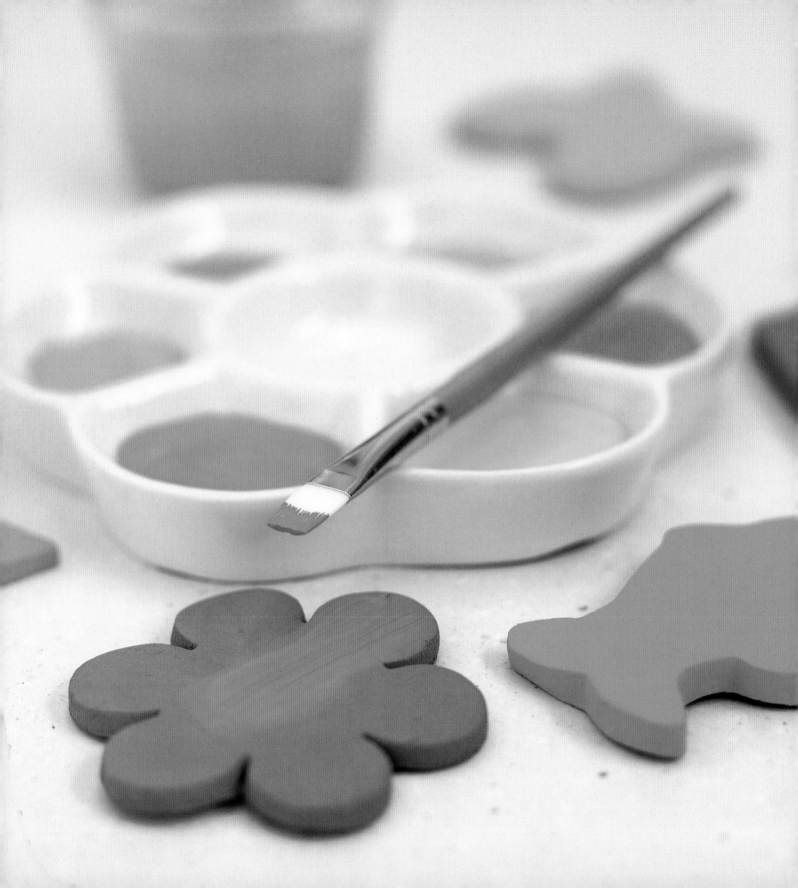

introduction

If you have kids, you'll know that they love pottering around with paint, scissors, and glue. As well as providing an outlet for their creativity, crafting has educational benefits too. Modeling, cutting, and painting will help develop hand-eye coordination, while learning to follow simple instructions is an important skill. And craft activities keep kids occupied and happy without having to resort to the TV or computer screen.

What Shall We Do Today? is packed with projects especially designed to appeal to children aged between 3 and 10 years. The book is arranged by season, and each section is full of ideas for crafting activities. There are suggestions for handmade gifts, things to grow, and pretty decorations to make—absorbing projects that will keep kids entertained on long summer days and rainy afternoons alike. There's something for everyone—modeling, papier mâché, tie-dye, and much, much more. And each project is accompanied by step-by-step photographs that simplify the technique and make the project foolproof.

If your kids are keen crafters, it's a good idea to put together a craft cupboard. Stock it with basic crafting materials—glue, adhesive tape, paper and card, pencils and paint—and add scraps of gift wrap or fabric, bits of ribbon, paper doilies, glitter pens, and so on. Then, when your kids want to get crafting, they'll have everything they need ready at hand.

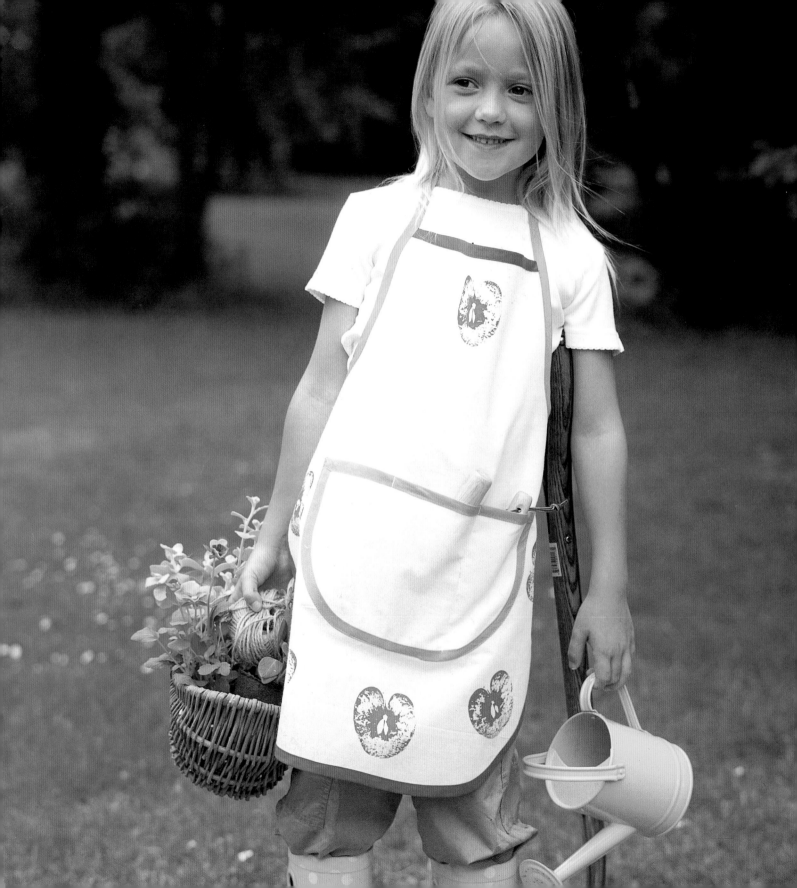

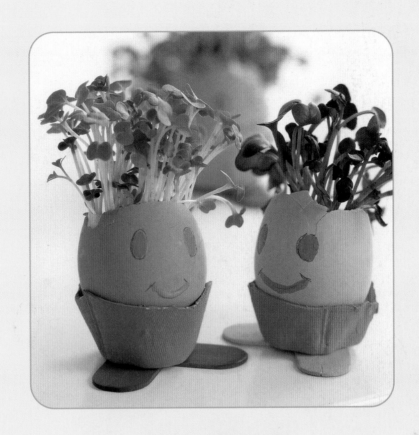

spring

valentine's day card

This three-dimensional Valentine's Day card features hearts cut from decorative handmade paper. Tissue paper and paper doilies would also make pretty hearts for the card. Use pinking shears and decorative scissors (available from craft stores) to cut the paper, and finish with a ribbon bow.

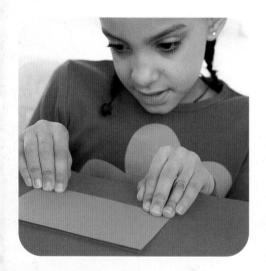

1 DRAW HEARTS For the card, you need three heart shapes in decreasing sizes. Fold three pieces of decorative paper in half and press the crease flat. Draw half a heart shape in three different sizes onto each folded piece of decorative paper. Alternatively, you could trace the heart templates on page 152 onto paper and cut them out. Place the templates on your chosen paper and draw round them before cutting them out.

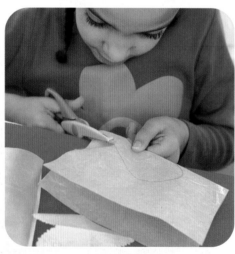

2 CUT OUT HEARTS Use the decorative cutting scissors or pinking shears to cut all the way around the edges of the heart motif, and then open it out flat. Cut out two smaller heart shapes in the same way. If you wish, you can cut out more hearts in graduating sizes to make an even more decorative card.

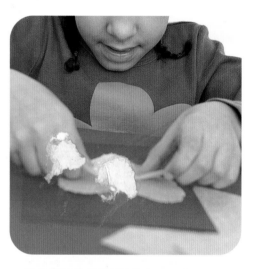

3 LAYER HEARTS Apply a line of glue down the center of the back of the largest heart, stick to the middle of the card and press flat. Apply glue to the center back of the smaller heart and glue to the first heart shape on the card. Apply the smallest heart in the same way. Allow the glue to dry.

WHAT YOU WILL NEED

- selection of decorative paper (scraps of wrapping paper are ideal)
- blank greeting cards (or pieces of card stock folded in half)
- pinking shears or other decorative cutting scissors
- glue
- ribbon for bows
- pencil
- plain paper for template (if using)

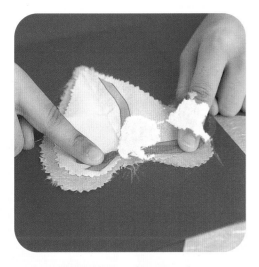

4 FINISHING Using sheer organza or velvet ribbon, cut a bow and trim the ends diagonally to prevent the ribbon fraying. Apply a small dot of glue to the central knot of the bow and stick to the heart. Leave to dry. A matching ribbon looks pretty stuck onto the back of the envelope flap, too.

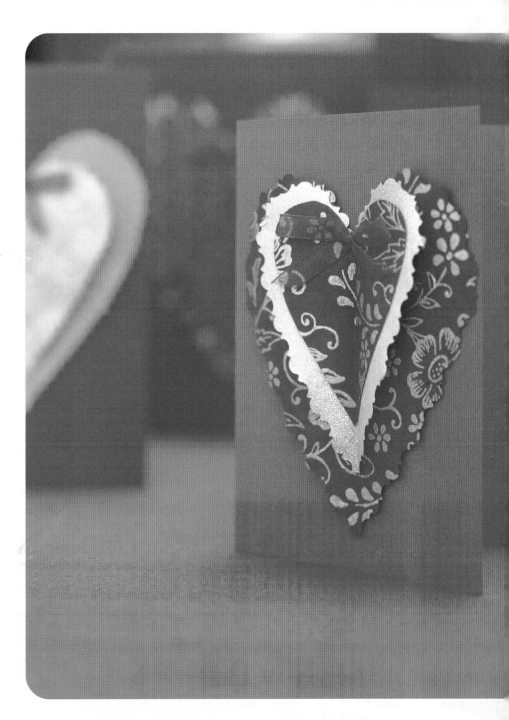

mother's day gift

This dainty decorated bowl is perfect for a Mother's Day gift. It uses the traditional papier mâché technique combined with layers of white glue and plastic wrap, which means that the bowl can be created with fewer layers of paper to give a more delicate appearance.

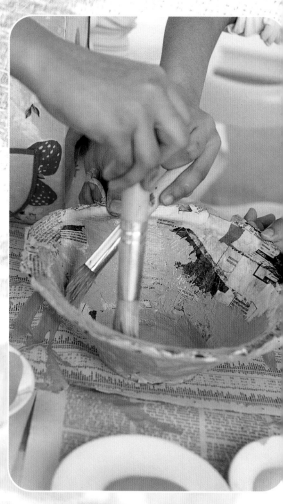

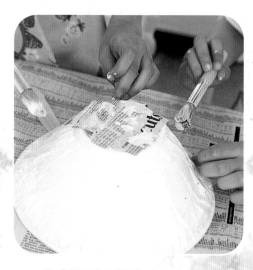

1 COVER BOWL Place your bowl mold upside down on a flat surface and cover it with a layer of plastic wrap. Tear the newspaper into strips. Paint over the plastic wrap with a thin layer of white glue, then carefully apply the first layer of paper. Repeat this process until you have built up four layers of paper. Leave to dry overnight.

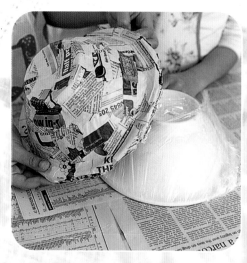

2 LIFT OFF PAPIER MÂCHÉ BOWL When it is completely dry, gently ease the papier mâché bowl away from the ceramic bowl and remove the plastic wrap. You can tidy the edges of the bowl with scissors, if desired.

3 PAINT THE BOWL Using a thick paintbrush, paint the bowl inside and out with the main color. Allow to dry, then apply a further coat of paint. Leave to dry before applying the decoration to the bowl.

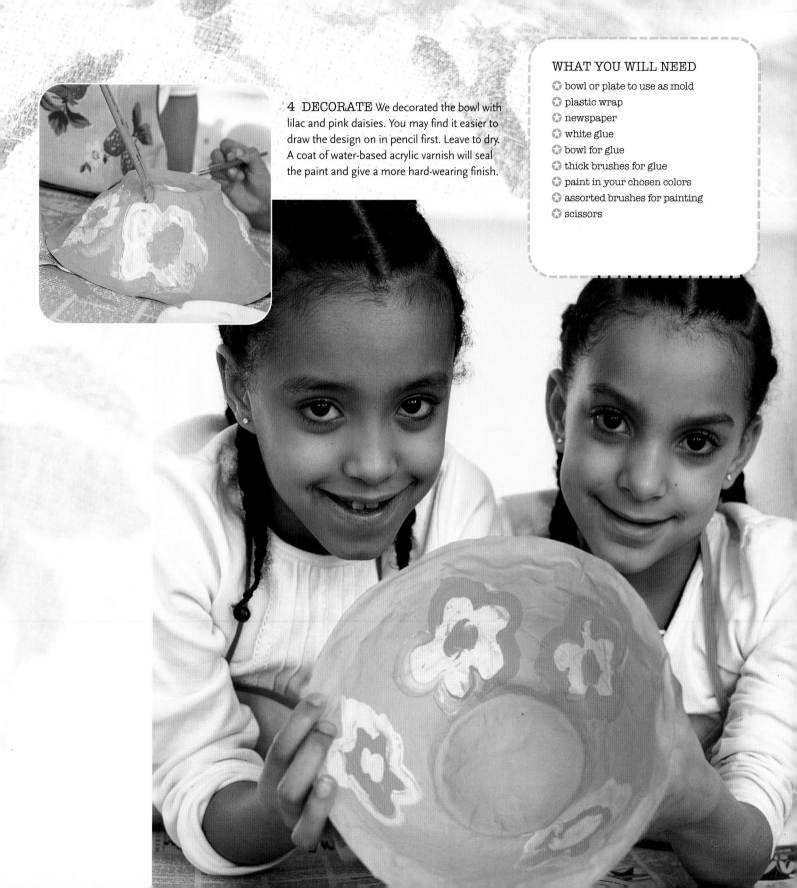

4 DECORATE We decorated the bowl with lilac and pink daisies. You may find it easier to draw the design on in pencil first. Leave to dry. A coat of water-based acrylic varnish will seal the paint and give a more hard-wearing finish.

WHAT YOU WILL NEED

- ❁ bowl or plate to use as mold
- ❁ plastic wrap
- ❁ newspaper
- ❁ white glue
- ❁ bowl for glue
- ❁ thick brushes for glue
- ❁ paint in your chosen colors
- ❁ assorted brushes for painting
- ❁ scissors

paper windmills

Boys and girls alike will delight in making these colorful, old-fashioned windmills that twirl gaily in even the slightest breeze. Try making extra ones and stick them into flowerpots for fun party decorations.

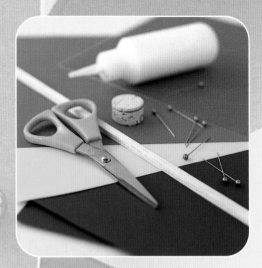

1 CHOOSE COLORS Choose the colors of paper you are going to use to make the windmill. We used bold green, blue, and yellow, but soft pastels or hot pink and zingy orange look great too.

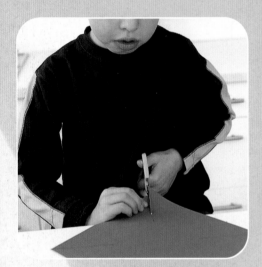

2 GLUE AND CUT Apply a thin layer of glue to one sheet of paper. Lay the other sheet on top and press flat. Rub gently, making sure there are no wrinkles or air bubbles between the two sheets. Allow the glue to dry. Now, from the corner of each square, cut a line approximately 4in/10cm long toward the center of the paper.

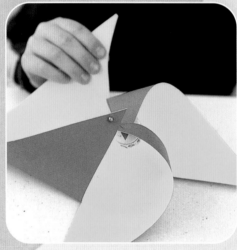

3 FORM BLADES With the paper in front of you, gently bend every other point of the paper into the center of the paper. Hold in place with your fingers until all four corners are folded into the center.

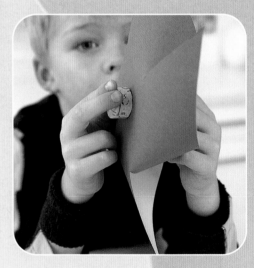

4 SECURE WITH PIN Push a pin through the center, making sure it goes through all four corners. It is advisable for an adult to do this. Push the pin into a cork. Using strong glue, attach the stick to the back of the cork, and allow to dry. Glue on a disc of card to hide the head of the pin, if desired.

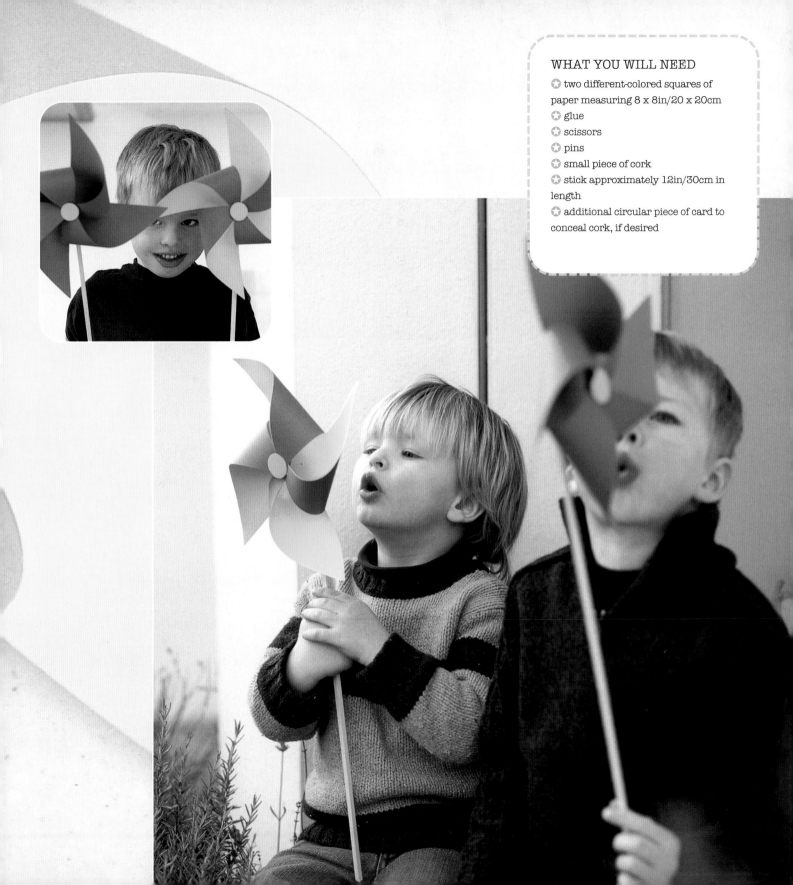

WHAT YOU WILL NEED

✪ two different-colored squares of paper measuring 8 x 8in/20 x 20cm
✪ glue
✪ scissors
✪ pins
✪ small piece of cork
✪ stick approximately 12in/30cm in length
✪ additional circular piece of card to conceal cork, if desired

weaving

Weaving is fun for most ages except the very young. The technique is easy to accomplish and can be applied to both two- and three-dimensional projects. Children will enjoy weaving cushions or bags from ribbons, or pen pots or boxes from colored pipe-cleaners.

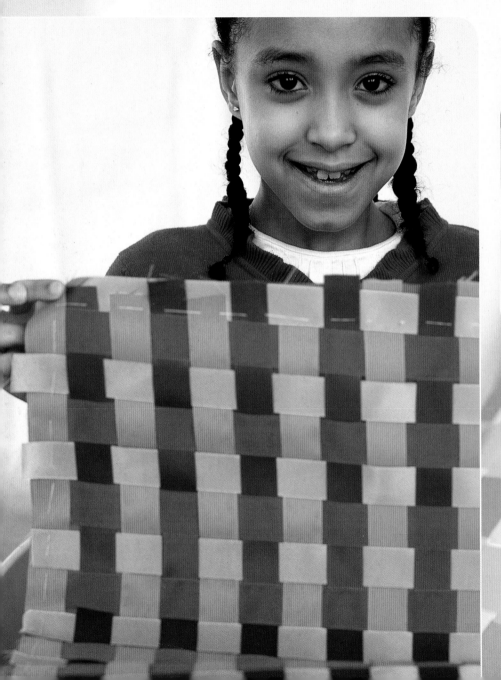

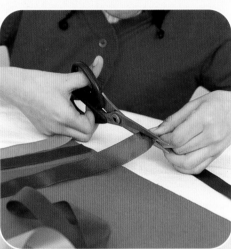

1 CUT THE RIBBON Cut the ribbon into 18in/45cm lengths and divide into separate piles by color. We used brightly colored satin ribbon, although you could substitute pretty pastels or fabric cut into narrow strips with a pair of pinking shears.

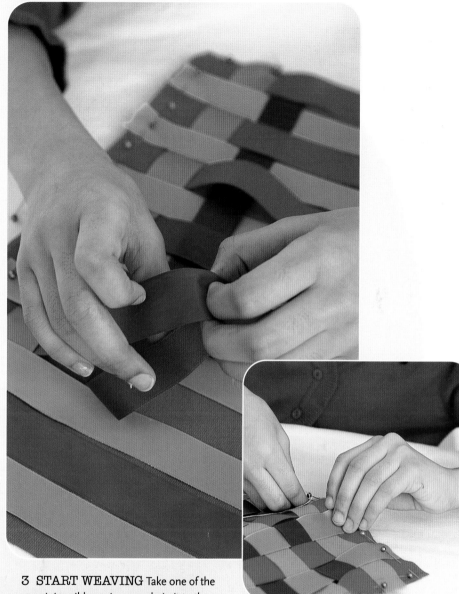

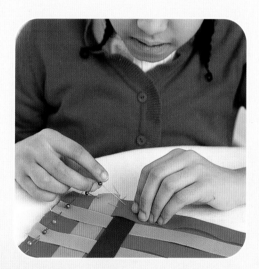

2 PIN ALONG EDGE Carefully arrange the ribbon lengths down one side of the fabric square, alternating two different colors. Pin the ribbons in place using one pin per length of ribbon to hold them firmly in place during weaving.

3 START WEAVING Take one of the remaining ribbon pieces and pin it to the adjacent side of the fabric square. Thread the ribbon over the first piece of ribbon and under the next and repeat until you reach the other side of the fabric square. Pin in place. Repeat with the other ribbon color until the weaving is finished. Pin each piece of ribbon in place to stop it from slipping.

4 STITCH TO BASE Use a needle and thread to sew neatly all the way around the four sides of the woven ribbon square, stitching it firmly to the backing square.

printed apron

This fun gardening apron is printed with a design of apples, created using the traditional potato-printing method. The outline of the apple makes a simple, bold motif on the fabric. Use a store-bought apron or make your own from calico and colorful bias binding.

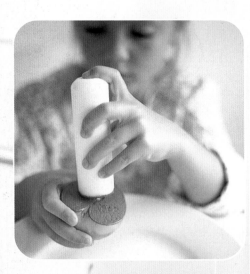

1 APPLY PAINT TO STAMP
Ask a grown-up to cut the apple in half. Blot it with a paper towel to remove excess moisture. Squirt some paint in a saucer, dip the roller in the paint, and blot on side of plate to remove excess paint. Apply paint to the apple.

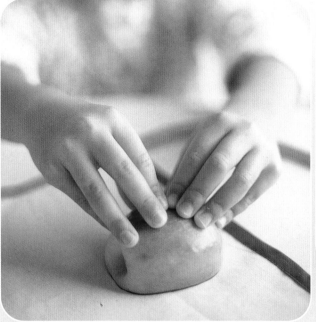

2 STAMP DESIGN ON APRON
Carefully place the apple cut-side down on the apron and press down firmly to make the imprint. Use a slight rocking motion to make sure the paint has been applied to the whole area, but be careful not to smudge the print.

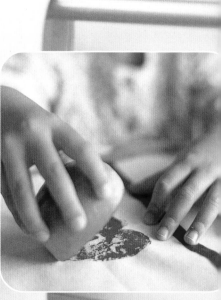

3 FINISHING Using the roller, apply more paint to the apple, then repeat the design all around the apron, as desired. Allow the paint to dry thoroughly, then iron the apron to seal the paint (following the manufacturer's instructions).

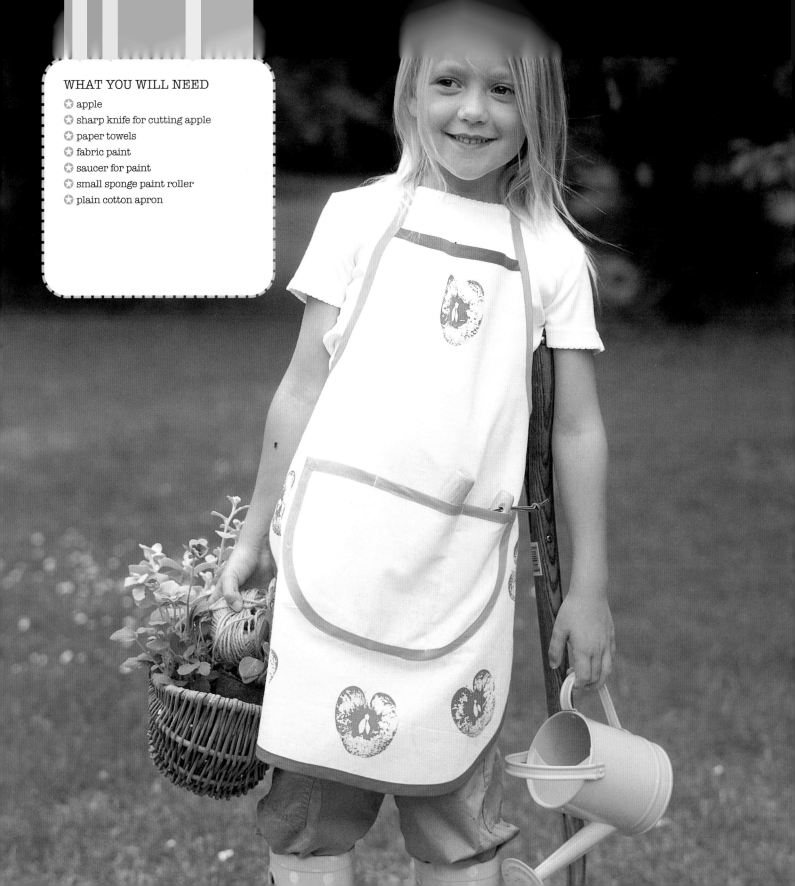

WHAT YOU WILL NEED

- ⭐ apple
- ⭐ sharp knife for cutting apple
- ⭐ paper towels
- ⭐ fabric paint
- ⭐ saucer for paint
- ⭐ small sponge paint roller
- ⭐ plain cotton apron

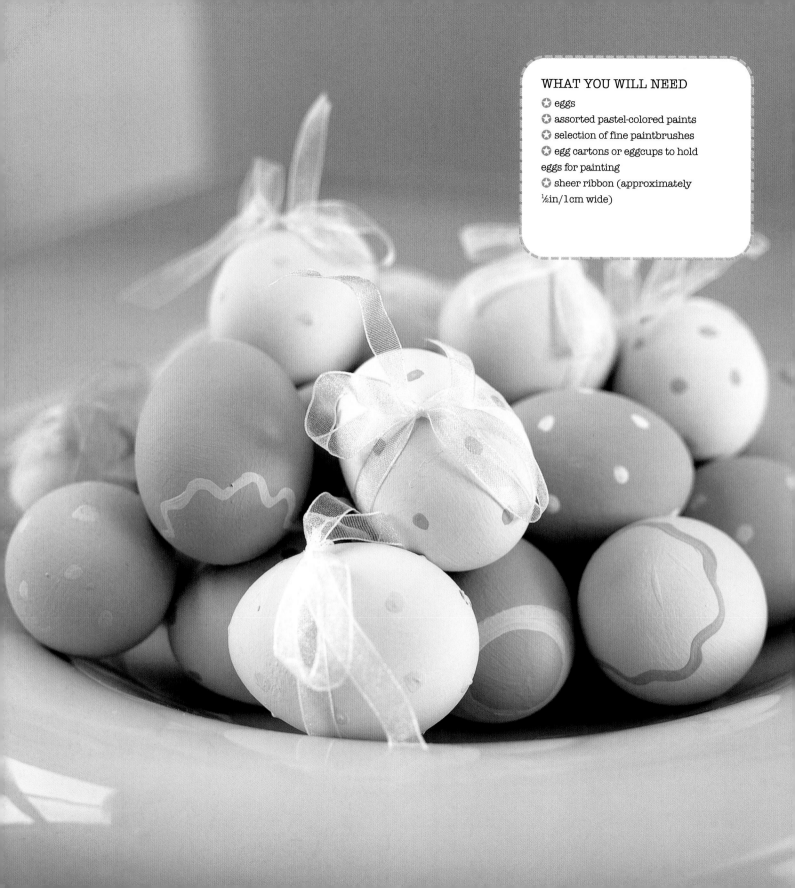

WHAT YOU WILL NEED

✿ eggs
✿ assorted pastel-colored paints
✿ selection of fine paintbrushes
✿ egg cartons or eggcups to hold
eggs for painting
✿ sheer ribbon (approximately
½in/1cm wide)

painted eggs

Real eggs painted in soft pastel colors and tied with sheer organza ribbons make a very simple but effective display for Easter. Older children may like to blow the eggs first, but if smaller children are involved, it is easier simply to boil the eggs before painting and decorating.

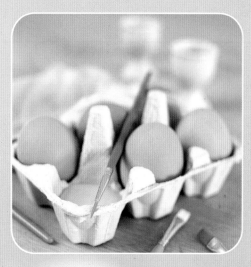

1 TAKE THE EGGS Select the eggs and boil the required number for decorating. Allow the eggs to cool completely before you start decorating them. You may like to cut up egg cartons to hold the eggs while you are painting them.

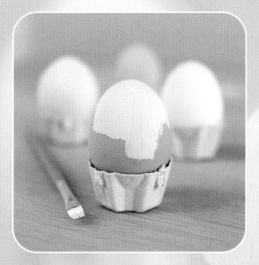

2 PAINT EGGS Paint the eggs in the chosen base color and allow them to dry completely. You may need to apply a second coat for good coverage. Allow to dry before adding any further decoration.

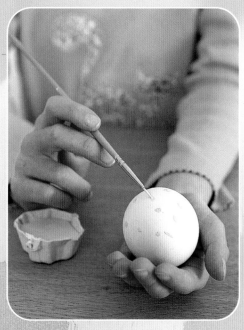

3 ADD DECORATION Use a fine paintbrush to add dots, swirls, and stripes in a contrasting colored paint, then allow to dry thoroughly. It is easier to paint one half of the egg first, then to leave it to dry before completing the other side, to prevent the paint from smudging.

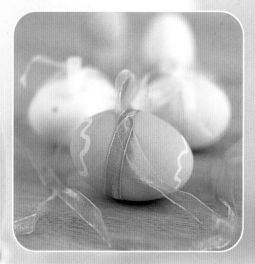

4 FINISHING Cut lengths of sheer ribbon and tie one around each egg, finishing with a bow. Group the eggs together in a bowl or on a glass cakestand to create a decorative Easter display.

burlap tote

Use natural burlap to make this practical yet pretty garden tote, then use it to hold garden tools, seeds, plant labels, and other gardening essentials. With its simple but striking painted design of peas and carrots, it would make a great gift for a keen gardener, too.

WHAT YOU WILL NEED

✪ 12in/30cm burlap fabric (approximately 54in/137cm wide)
✪ scissors
✪ fabric paint in green and orange
✪ fine paintbrush
✪ pins
✪ lime green and brown embroidery thread
✪ needle
✪ iron-on fusible interlining

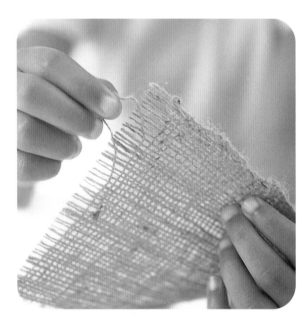

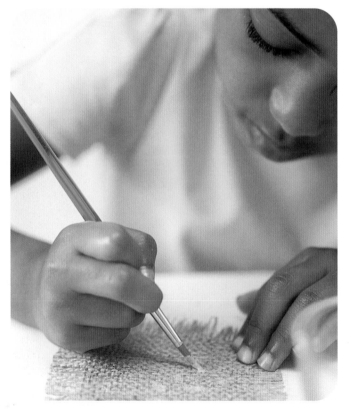

1 CUT OUT FABRIC Cut a piece of burlap measuring 22 x 7in/55 x 18cm for the main bag, four 4 x 4in/10 x 10cm squares of burlap for the pockets, one oval with a diameter of 8 x 5in/20 x 14cm, plus two lengths measuring 10 x 3in/25 x 8cm for the handles. Use the selvage of the fabric for the top of the pockets and for one of the longer sides of the handle sections to prevent fraying.

2 DECORATE POCKETS On the remaining three edges of each pocket, carefully pull away strands of burlap to fray the edges about ¹/₂in/1cm from each side. Use a brush to paint a design on the pockets. Fix the paint according to the manufacturer's instructions.

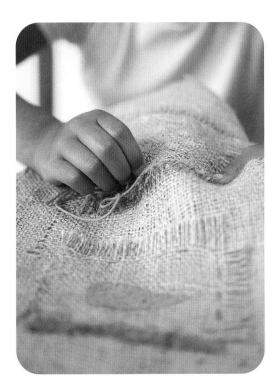

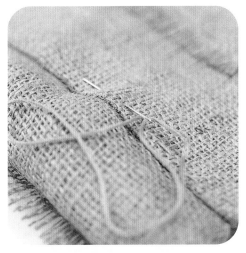

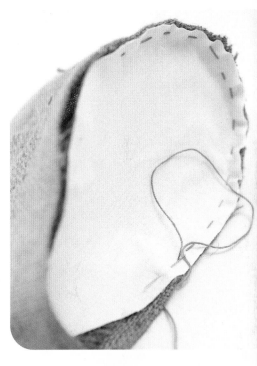

3 ATTACH POCKETS Take the length of the large burlap rectangle (allowing $\frac{1}{2}$in/1cm at each end for the seams) and pin the pockets in place at evenly spaced intervals. Using green embroidery thread, make small running stitches to attach the pockets to the bag, leaving the selvage open at the top.

4 SEW SEAM Fold the piece of burlap with right sides facing, and stitch the sides of the bag together $\frac{1}{2}$in/1cm from the edge. Turn to right side and press both layers of the seam to one side. Using brown embroidery thread, stitch a row of running stitches along this seam to prevent the edges from fraying.

5 STITCH BASE TO BAG Iron the fusible interlining to one side of the burlap oval (it is advisable for an adult to do this). Now, with right sides facing, stitch the oval to the bag. Whipstitch around the raw edges to prevent them from fraying.

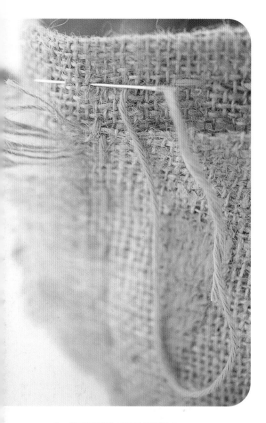

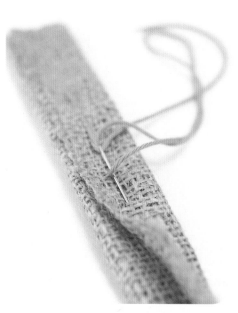

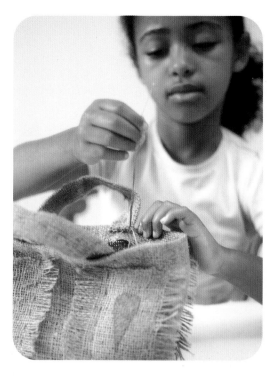

6 STITCH TOP HEM Turn the top of the bag 1½in/3cm to the inside and press flat with an iron, if necessary. Use lime green embroidery thread and running stitch to secure in place.

7 MAKE HANDLES Lay the two handle sections flat, turn the top and bottom over by ½in/1cm and press. Fold the long edges 1in/2cm to the inside, making sure that the selvage edge is on top. Use running stitch to hold in place.

8 FINISHING The handles should be positioned along the sides of the oval base shape, just above the pockets. Stitch the ends of the handles to the inside of the bag, spacing them approximately 5in/12cm apart. Use whipstitch to hold the handles securely in place.

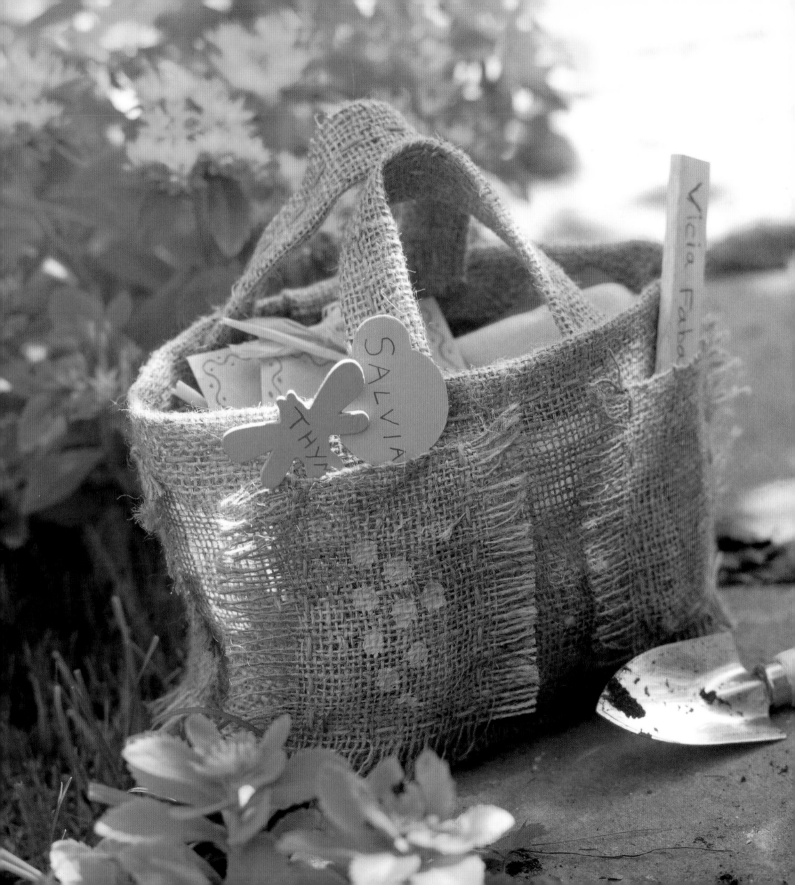

gingerbread people

Don't just make people—look out for cutters in the shape of a princess, a pony, teddy bear, or Santa. Decorate them with chocolate chips, M&Ms® or raisins.

1 Ask an adult to help you preheat the oven to 325°F/160°C. Grease several baking trays with soft butter, using a piece of paper towel.

2 Set a strainer over a large bowl. Tip the flour, salt, and ground ginger into the strainer and sift into the bowl. Add the sugar and mix in with a wooden spoon. Make a hollow in the center of the dry ingredients.

3 Put the butter and syrup into a small saucepan. Ask an adult to help you melt the butter and syrup gently over very low heat—warm the pan just enough to melt the ingredients. Don't let the mixture become hot.

4 Carefully pour the melted mixture into the hollow in the dry ingredients.

5 Crack the egg into a small bowl and break up with a fork.

6 Pour the egg into the hollow on top of the melted mixture. Now mix all the ingredients together with a wooden spoon. As soon as the dough starts to come together, put your hands into the bowl and start to push the barely warm dough together. If the dough is too hot to handle, wait for it to cool.

7 As soon as the dough has come together into a ball and is no longer crumbly, tip it out of the bowl and onto a work surface lightly dusted with flour.

8 With a rolling pin, gently roll out the dough into a large rectangle about ¼in/5mm thick.

9 Cut out figures with your cutters, then transfer them carefully to the prepared baking trays with a large spatula. Don't worry if their limbs or heads fall off—just press them back together again. Space the figures well apart, because they will spread in the oven. Gather all the trimmings into a ball, then roll out and cut more figures as before.

10 Decorate the figures with raisins, silver balls, or M&Ms®. Ask an adult to help you bake the figures—they will take about 15 minutes until golden brown. Watch them carefully, because they can easily burn.

11 Ask an adult to help you carefully remove the trays from the oven and leave them on a heatproof work surface to cool for 5 minutes. This lets the soft biscuit mixture become hard. When the figures are firm, gently lift them onto a wire rack, using a spatula. Let them cool completely.

12 Store in an airtight container and eat within 1 week.

WHAT YOU WILL NEED

- 2⅓ cups/350g self-rising flour
- a pinch of salt
- 1 tablespoon ground ginger
- 1 cup/200g superfine sugar
- 1 stick/115g unsalted butter
- ¼ cup/85g light corn syrup
- 1 large egg

TO DECORATE

- 2 baking sheets
- shaped pastry cutters
- raisins
- edible silver balls
- M&Ms®

makes approximately 14 figures, each 5in/12cm long

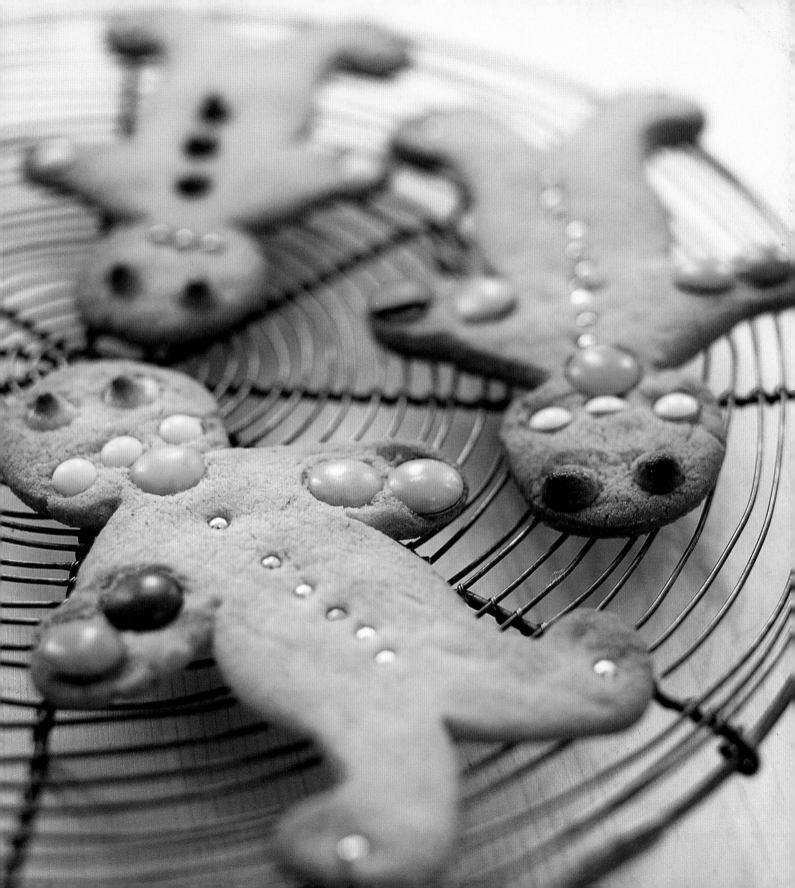

pompoms

Old-fashioned pompoms are so easy to make and are a great way of using up left-over wool. They can be made in a variety of sizes and used to create toys, including cute kittens or fluffy chicks for Easter, as well as fun jewelry and decorations.

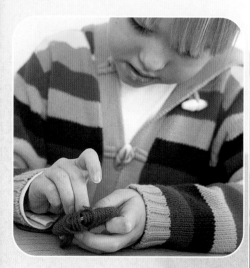

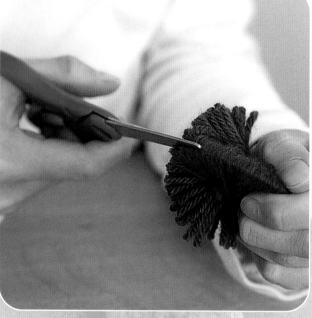

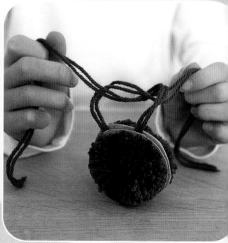

1 WIND THE WOOL Trace the pompom disc template on page 152 onto paper and cut it out. Place it on a piece of cardboard and draw round it. Repeat. Cut out two discs. Start to wind wool around the two discs. When the first ball of wool is finished, tie the end of the ball to the beginning of a new one. Continue winding the wool until the disc is completely covered.

2 CUT AROUND THE OUTSIDE
When the winding process is complete, hold the pompom discs securely in one hand, then cut all around the edges of the wool using scissors. The wool will come away and look like fringing at this point, and it is important that the two discs are firmly held together.

3 SECURE THE WOOL Cut two lengths of wool approximately 8in/20cm long and thread them between the two cardboard discs. Pull together tightly and tie in a knot. It is a good idea to tie several knots so that the wool is very secure.

YOU WILL NEED
- ✪ pencil
- ✪ scissors
- ✪ cardboard for pompom discs
- ✪ assorted balls of wool

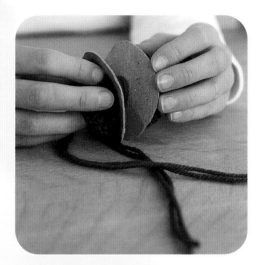

4 PULL APART AND FINISH
Gently pull away the cardboard discs from the pompom. If it proves difficult to remove them, just cut them off. Trim any excess bits of wool and fluff the pompom ball to give it a nice plump round shape.

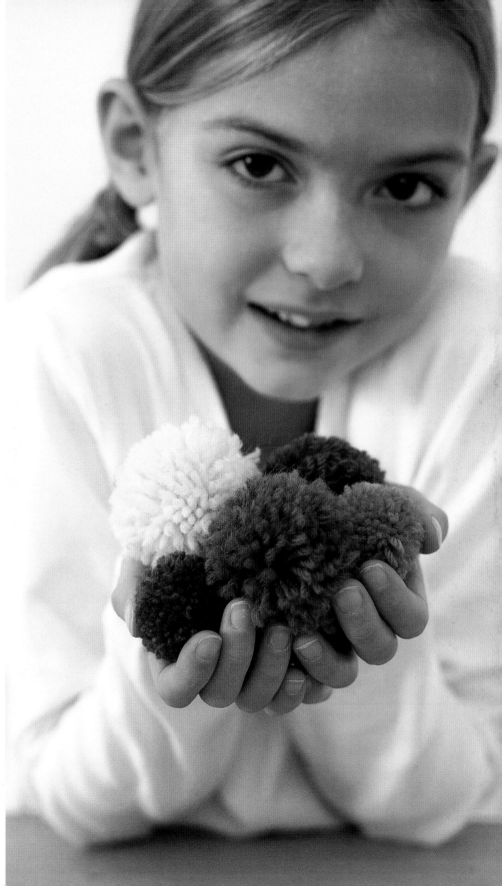

crazy eggheads

Creating these cute eggheads is really easy and fun. Fill them with cotton balls scattered with fast-growing seed, then sit back and watch the hair grow. Once the cress has sprouted and grown, give the "hair" a trim and add the yummy sprouts to your lunchtime sandwiches!

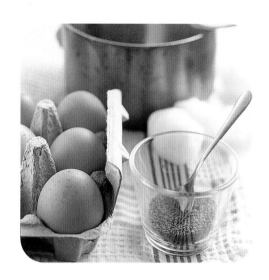

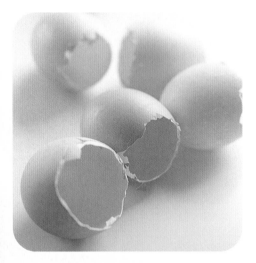

1 **PREPARE EGGS** Remove the top from a hard-cooked egg by gently tapping around the outside of the shell with a knife (make a hole that is large enough for you to extract the egg). Scoop out the egg with a teaspoon.

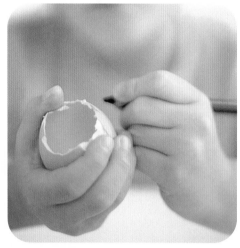

2 **DRAW ON FACE** Hold the shell gently in one hand, and draw a face on the outside with a pencil. Don't press too hard, or you might break the shell.

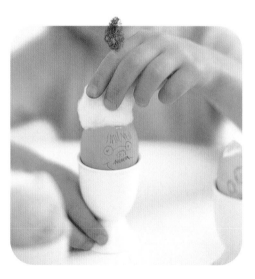

3 **ADD COTTON WOOL** Gently push a cotton ball into the bottom of the eggshell. Pour in some water and allow the cotton to soak it up.

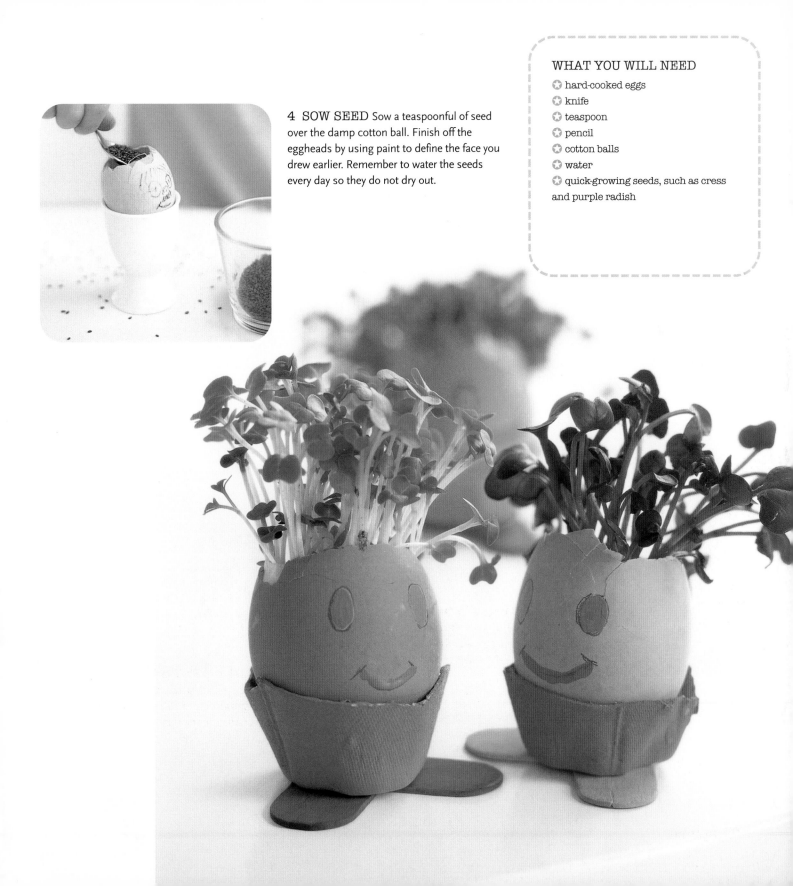

4 SOW SEED Sow a teaspoonful of seed over the damp cotton ball. Finish off the eggheads by using paint to define the face you drew earlier. Remember to water the seeds every day so they do not dry out.

WHAT YOU WILL NEED

✪ hard-cooked eggs
✪ knife
✪ teaspoon
✪ pencil
✪ cotton balls
✪ water
✪ quick-growing seeds, such as cress and purple radish

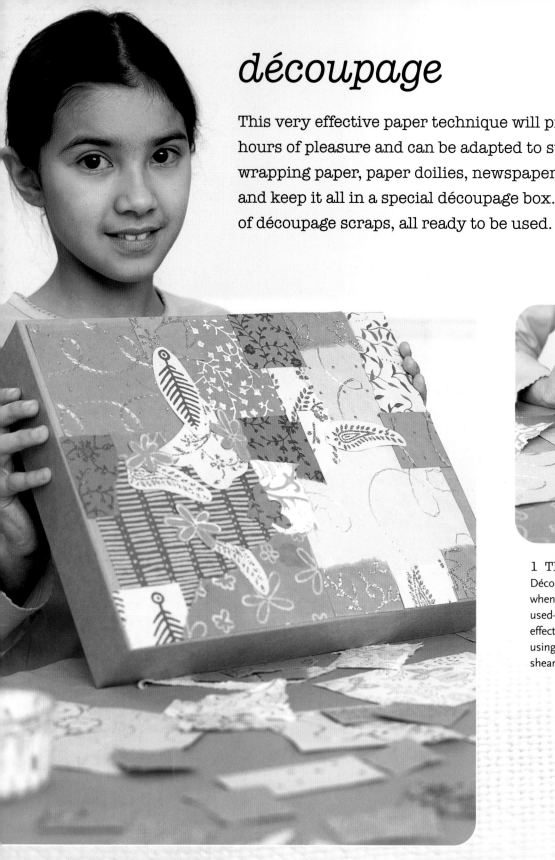

découpage

This very effective paper technique will provide children with hours of pleasure and can be adapted to suit most ages. Collect wrapping paper, paper doilies, newspapers, and magazine cuttings and keep it all in a special découpage box. You can also buy books of découpage scraps, all ready to be used.

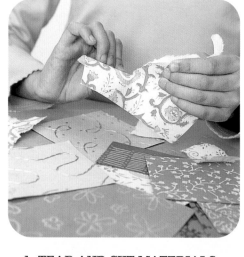

1 TEAR AND CUT MATERIALS

Découpage looks particularly effective when both cut and torn pieces of paper are used—the ragged edges add to the layered effect. For added interest, you could also try using decorative scissors and pinking shears to cut some of the paper.

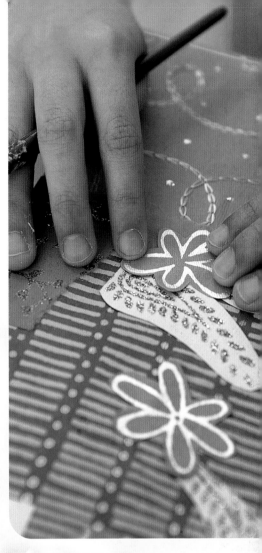

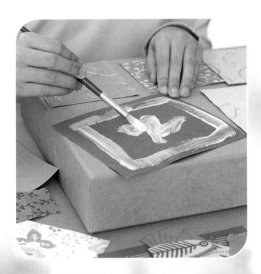

2 GLUE ON Start by sticking on larger pieces of paper to cover the box completely. This provides a good background for the smaller pieces of paper, which can be added later. Allow the glue to dry before applying the next layer of paper.

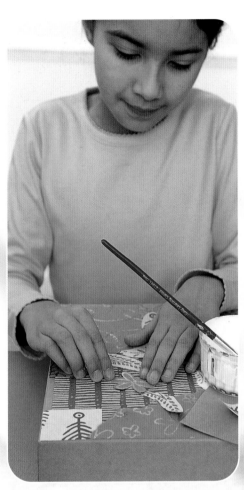

3 LAYER UPON LAYER When the first layer is dry, add smaller pieces of paper. We used torn pieces of paper as well as smaller squares to cover the box. Allow some drying time between layers, so the wet glue does not cause the layer beneath to peel away.

4 FINISHING Finish the découpage with smaller shapes such as flowers or leaves cut from wrapping paper. It may be easier to use a fine paintbrush to apply the glue to these smaller, more fiddly pieces of paper.

spring 33

paper flowers

Paper flowers are easy to make and are a great way of using up scraps of wrapping paper and tissue. Use pipe-cleaners to make stems and stand the flowers in vases made from plastic cups covered in tissue paper. Alternatively, use the flowers to make jewelry or to decorate handmade cards.

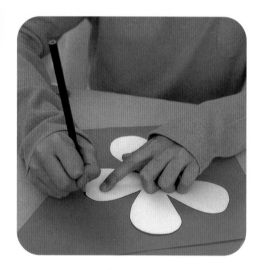

1 DRAW OUT FLOWER Trace the flower template on page 153 onto paper and cut it out. Draw around the template on colored card stock and cut out the flower shape carefully.

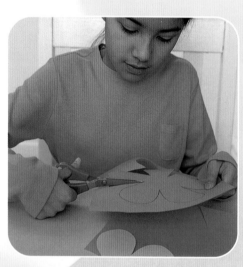

2 CUT OUT PETALS Layer the flowers by cutting out five petals from crêpe or tissue paper in a contrasting color. These petals can be glued on top of the flower to create a fuller effect.

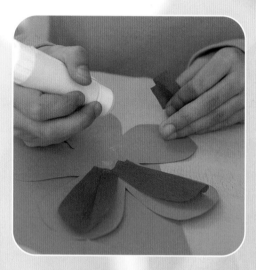

3 GLUE ON PETALS Fold a small pleat in the bottom end of each petal. Apply glue to the back of a petal and stick it to the center of the card flower. Repeat for each petal, then let the glue dry completely.

WHAT YOU WILL NEED

- ✪ paper for flower template
- ✪ pencil
- ✪ scissors
- ✪ colored card stock for the main flower shape and the flower centers
- ✪ colored tissue paper or crêpe paper
- ✪ stick of glue
- ✪ adhesive tape
- ✪ pipe-cleaners for the flower stems

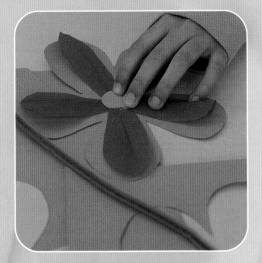

4 FINISHING Cut out a small circle of card, approximately 1in/2cm in diameter, and glue it to the center of the flower to cover the ends of the petals. Use a small piece of tape to attach a pipe-cleaner to the back of the flower to form a stem.

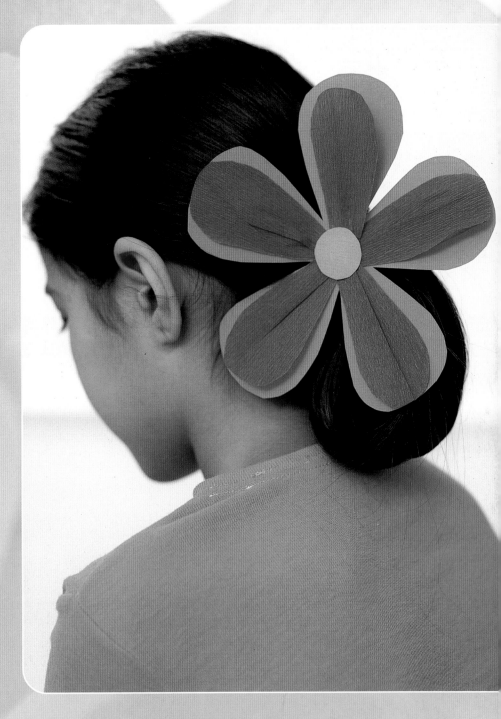

tin can windchime

Make a musical windchime using an old tin can and pretty glass beads, then hang it from a tree in the yard. The tin is pierced with small holes for fixing the hanging decorations, so it's important to ask an adult to do this before starting the project.

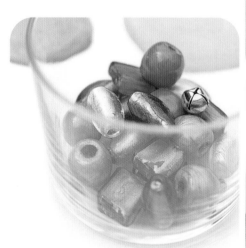

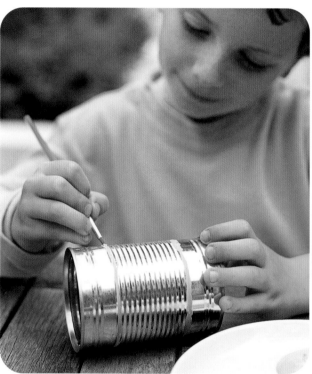

1 PIERCE HOLES Ask an adult to pierce the holes in the tin before you start. You need two holes either side of the open end of the tin for the hanging wire. On the bottom of the tin, pierce one hole in the center, four holes evenly spaced around the outside edge of the tin, and four holes evenly spaced around the central hole. Now use a fine paintbrush to paint four narrow stripes around the outside of the tin, using the ridges of the tin as an outline.

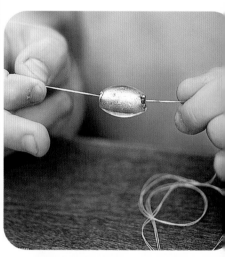

2 START THREADING Cut a length of thread 8in/20cm long and then attach one of the metal bells to the bottom, knotting it several times to secure. Begin threading four glass beads onto the string.

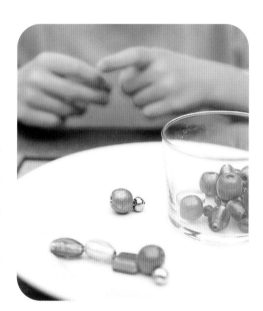

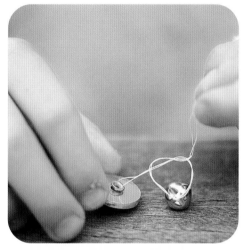

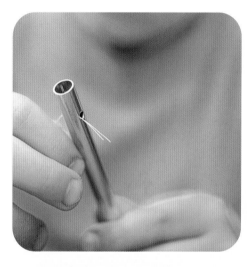

3 TIE ON BELLS Repeat until you have made four bead lengths. We used pretty colored glass beads, but you could use varnished wood beads for a more natural effect.

4 THREAD ON CLAPPER Take a length of thread approximately 8in/20cm long and attach a bell to the end. Knot securely in place. Thread on the metal clapper, so that it hangs from the bottom of the cotton, just above the bell.

5 THREAD ON CHIMES Cut a piece of thread approximately 12in/30cm long. Double it, and knot the ends. Now thread it through the hole in the tubular chime and pull through so that it forms a loop.

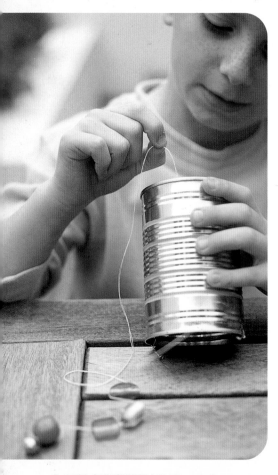

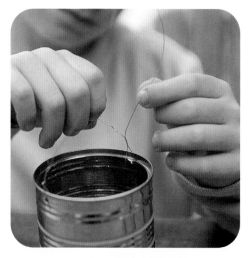

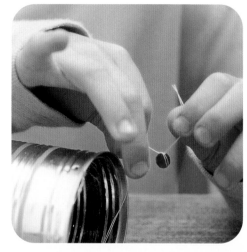

6 TIE ON THREAD The tubular chimes, clapper and beaded decorations are all attached to the inside of the tin by feeding the thread through the holes in the tin base and pulling through. The clapper must go through the central hole in the bottom of the tin and the tubular chimes around this. Finally, thread the beaded decorations through the outside holes.

7 FIX WIRE HANDLE Thread a 12in/30cm length of fine wire through the two holes punched in the sides of the top (open) end of the tin. Twist the wire around itself to secure in place. This is the loop from which to hang your windchime.

8 FINISHING Gather all the pieces of thread together, push the ends through a bead, and knot securely. The bead will prevent the pieces of thread slipping through the hole in the base.

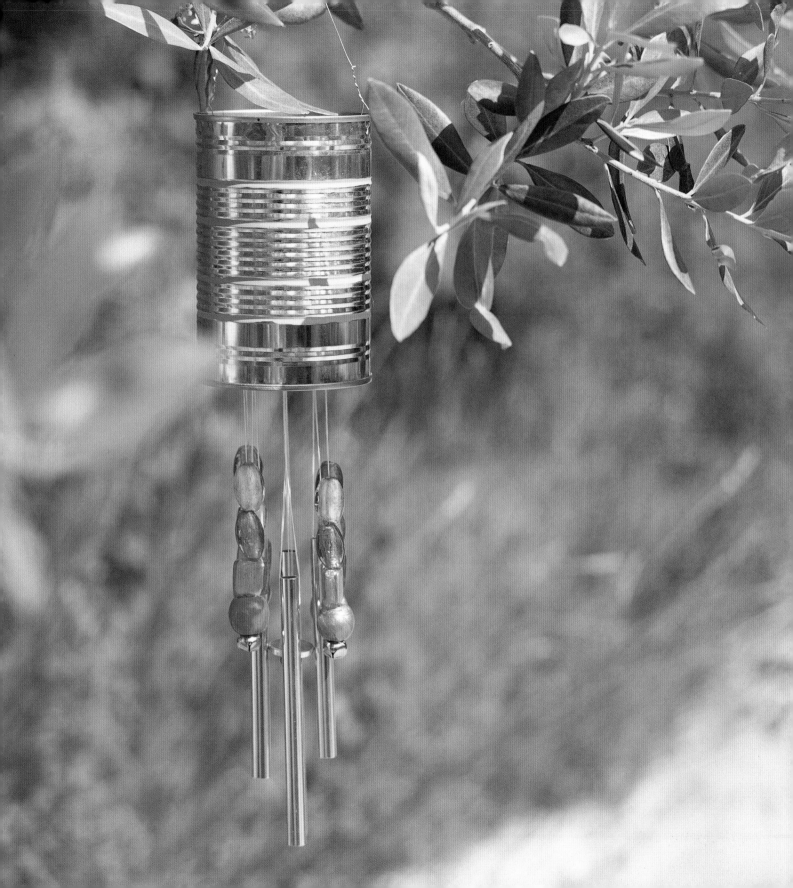

papier mâché dinosaur

Papier mâché is a really hands-on messy project, so make sure you have enough time to get the materials ready and to clear up afterwards! Kids love working with papier mâché due to its sloshy consistency and the fact it can be used to create fantastic three-dimensional objects.

WHAT YOU WILL NEED

- ✪ newspaper
- ✪ balloon
- ✪ bowl to support balloon
- ✪ thick brushes
- ✪ white glue
- ✪ bowl for glue
- ✪ aluminum foil (for the dinosaur's legs and head)
- ✪ masking tape
- ✪ cardboard
- ✪ two different colors of paint

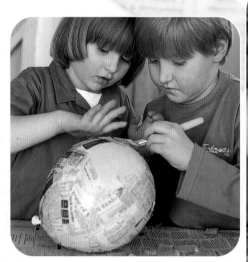

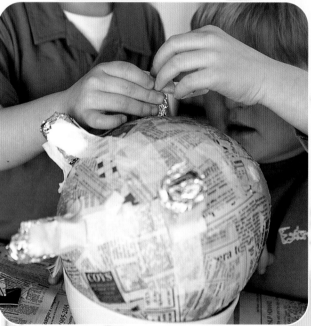

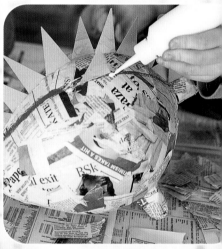

1 COVER BALLOON Tear the newspaper into strips and put to one side. Blow up the balloon and balance it on a bowl while you stick on the paper. Using a brush, apply glue all over the balloon. Cover with strips of newspaper. Repeat the process, building up layers of paper, until the balloon is thickly covered.

2 ADD LEGS AND HEAD We used ordinary aluminum foil rolled into short cylinder shapes to make the legs and head. Use masking tape to attach them to the balloon. Now apply a coat of glue to the legs and head and cover with strips of paper. Make sure that the strips overlap onto the body, so that the head and legs will be securely held in place once the glue has dried.

3 ADD SPINES Cut out triangles measuring approximately 1in/2cm wide and 10in/4cm high from the cardboard. Fold the bottom of the triangle at a ninety-degree angle and glue the flat part to the balloon. Form two lines to create the spines. When the glue is dry, apply another layer of paper to hold the spikes in place.

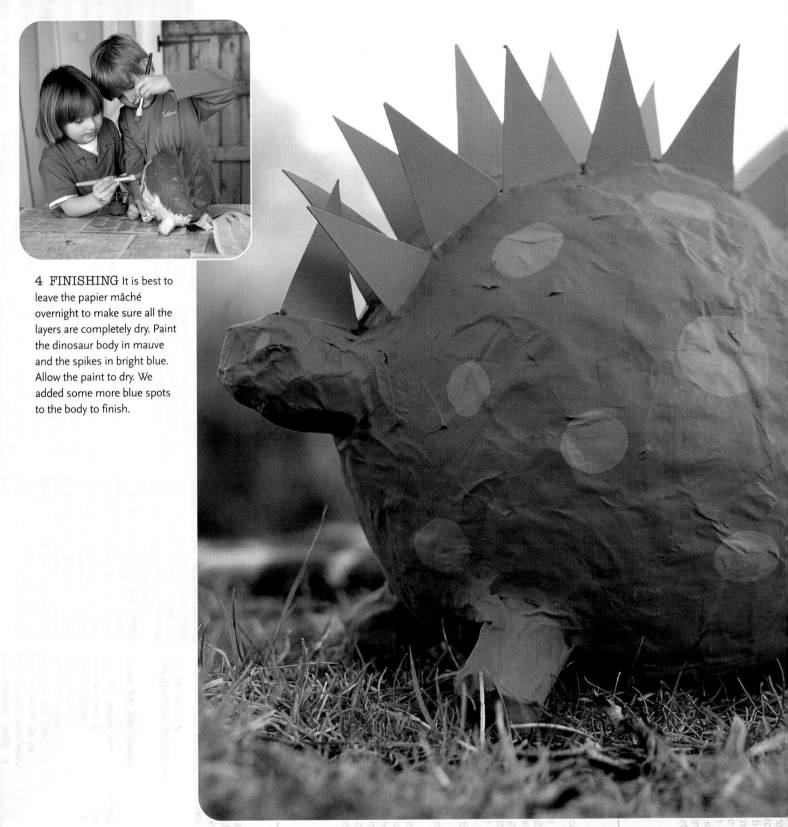

4 FINISHING It is best to leave the papier mâché overnight to make sure all the layers are completely dry. Paint the dinosaur body in mauve and the spikes in bright blue. Allow the paint to dry. We added some more blue spots to the body to finish.

wooden nesting box

Plain wooden nesting boxes can be decorated with wooden craft sticks and painted in soft pastel colors to create these fun boxes that will make a pretty addition to any tree or wall in the garden. Hang it in a sheltered spot, at least 6ft/2m above the ground.

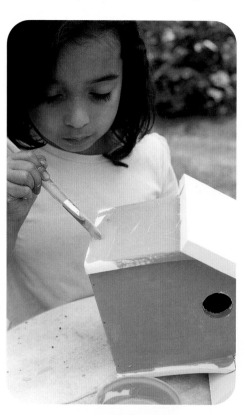

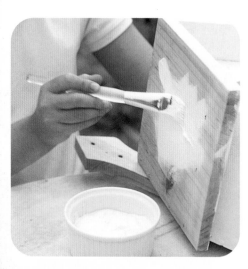

1 APPLY UNDERCOAT Use a large paintbrush to apply undercoat to the nesting box. Let it dry completely. Apply a second coat if necessary.

2 PAINT BASE COLOR Once the undercoat is dry, use a brush to apply the first coat of green paint to the nesting box. Do not paint over the undercoat on the roof, however. Apply a further coat of paint, if required, and allow to dry thoroughly.

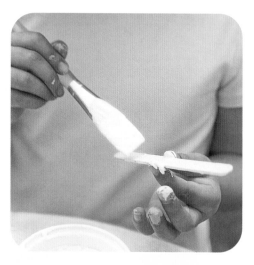

3 PAINT CRAFT STICKS Apply undercoat to one side and the edges of the standard-sized craft sticks, then leave them to dry. Next, paint the other sides of the sticks and leave them to dry. Once completely dry, paint the sticks cream.

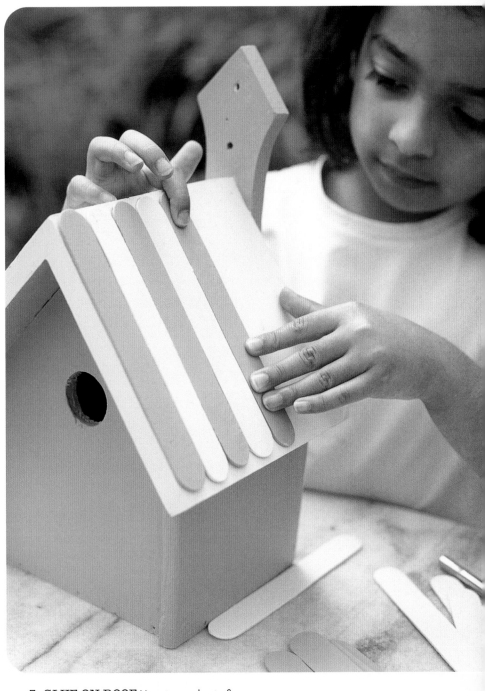

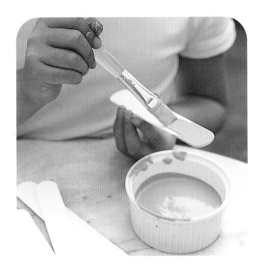

4 PAINT STICKS FOR ROOF Now take the larger craft sticks and divide them into two piles. Paint one pile of the larger craft sticks green, and the other ones cream. Allow to dry completely. Apply a further coat, if required.

5 GLUE ON ROOF Use strong glue to fix the large craft sticks to the roof. Glue them in alternate colors to create a striped effect, then leave the glue to dry.

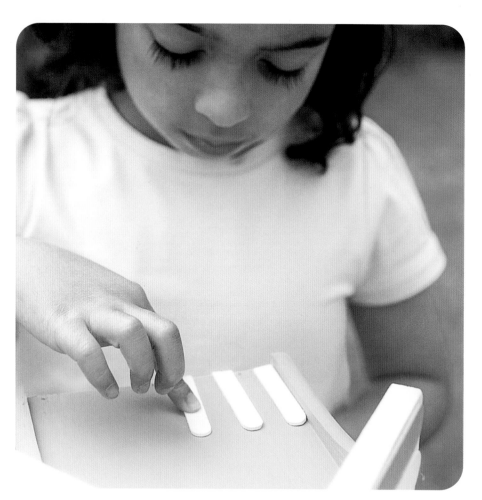

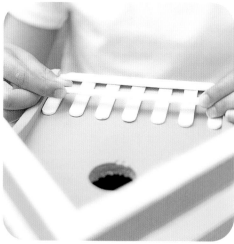

6 ATTACH PICKET FENCE Ask an adult to cut four of the smaller craft sticks in half for the picket fence. Lie them along the base of the front of the nesting box and glue them in an even row along this edge.

7 FINISHING Glue the two remaining smaller craft sticks across the halved sticks to complete the picket fence. Finish the nesting box with one or two coats of varnish to make it suitable for outdoor use.

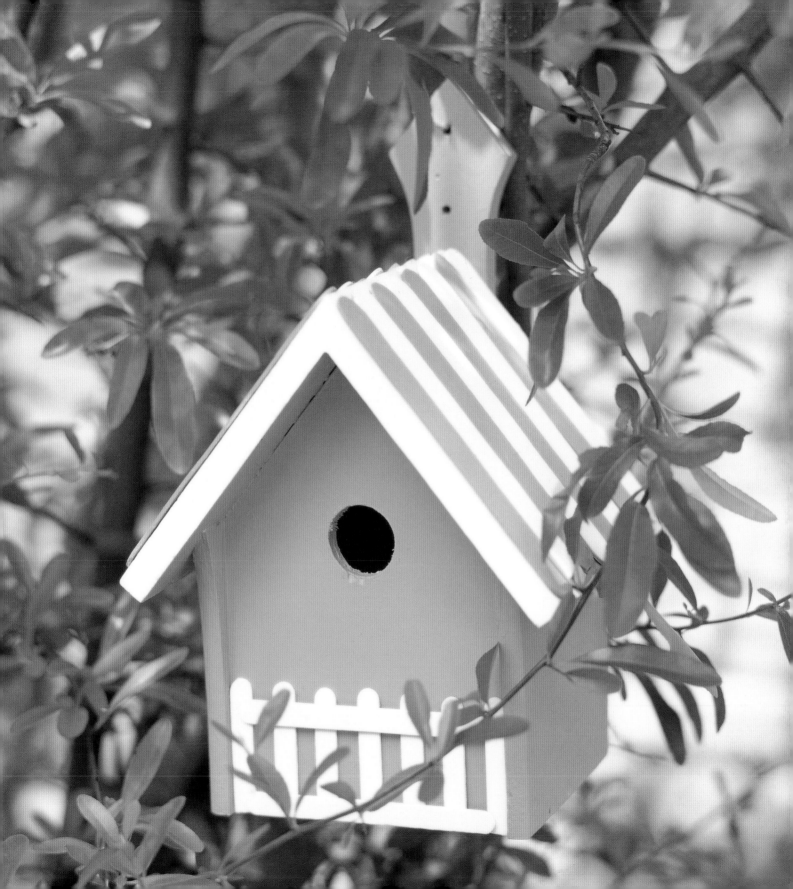

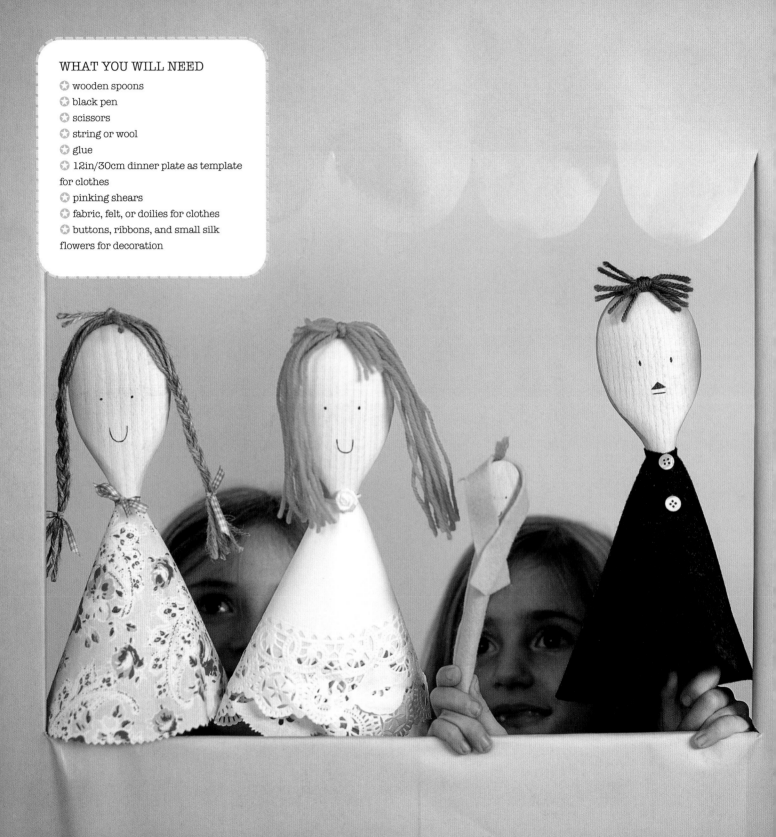

WHAT YOU WILL NEED

- ⭐ wooden spoons
- ⭐ black pen
- ⭐ scissors
- ⭐ string or wool
- ⭐ glue
- ⭐ 12in/30cm dinner plate as template for clothes
- ⭐ pinking shears
- ⭐ fabric, felt, or doilies for clothes
- ⭐ buttons, ribbons, and small silk flowers for decoration

wooden-spoon puppets

These classic spoon puppets have been made by children for years and provide hours of entertainment. Their outfits are made from semicircles of fabric or paper, while string or wool is used for the hair. We used a large cardboard box covered in wrapping paper to create a puppet theatre.

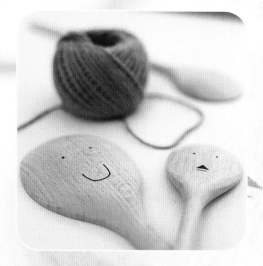

1 MAKING FACES Use a fine liner pen to draw the faces onto the wooden spoons. Let the child use his or her imagination and add rosy cheeks, noses, and eyebrows with colored pencils.

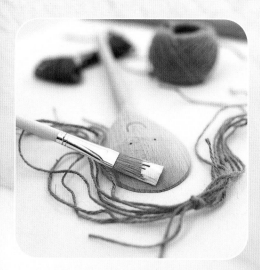

2 ADDING THE HAIR For plaited hair with a fringe, cut six lengths of string or wool measuring approximately 12in/30cm and two lengths measuring 3in/8cm. Knot the shorter pieces of string in the middle of the longer pieces to create the fringe effect. Alternatively, use ten 12in/30cm lengths for long loose hair, and six shorter 2½in/6cm lengths for the boy puppet's hair. Glue the hair to the top of the wooden spoon.

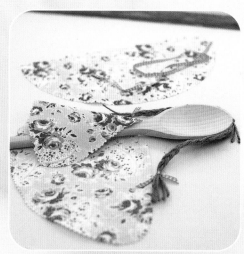

3 DRESSING UP Use a 12in/30cm dinner plate as a template. Place on your chosen fabric and draw round the edge with the black pen. Cut each circle out, then cut into two halves to create semicircular shapes. Use pinking shears to prevent the edges from fraying. Wrap the fabric around the neck of the spoon and glue in place. Add little buttons or ribbons to decorate.

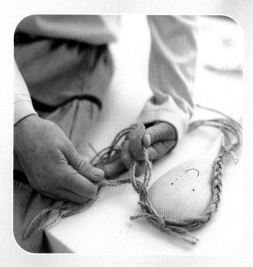

4 FINISHING Carefully plait the doll's hair and tie the ends with short lengths of colorful ribbon.

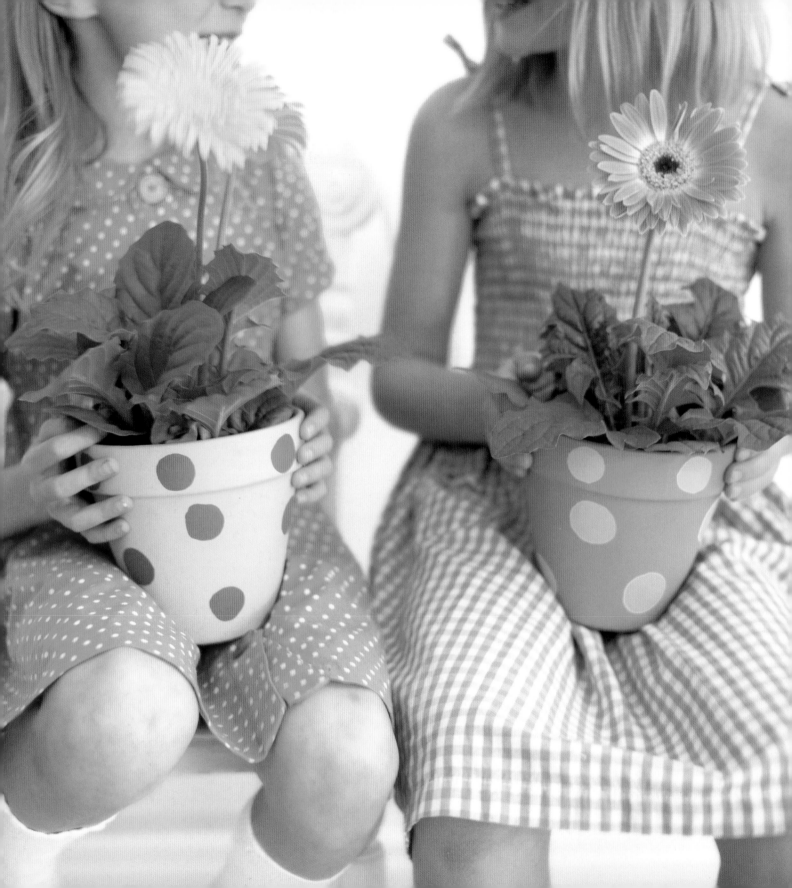

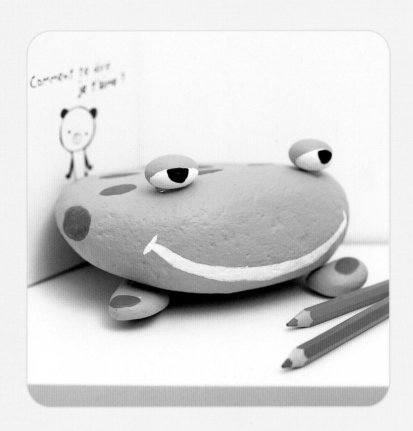

summer

funky fans

Create fans using brightly colored and decorative paper—sheets of wrapping paper are a perfect choice. Finished off with silk tassels, paper fans are easy to make, and are a great addition to the dress-up box.

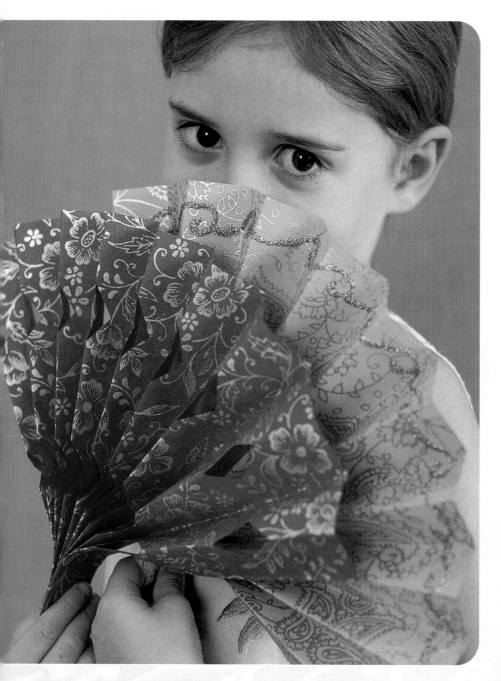

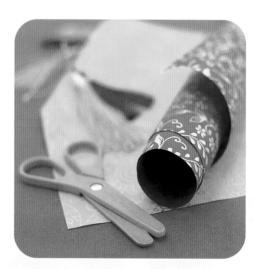

1 CUT OUT To make a paper fan, cut out one piece of paper measuring approximately 20 x 10in/50 x 25cm. The paper should not be too thin, or the finished fan will be floppy.

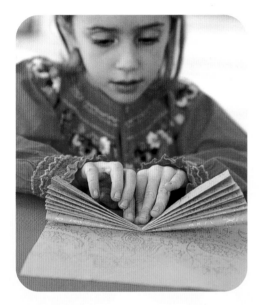

2 FOLD PAPER Place the sheet of paper flat on the table with the shortest edge in front of you. Starting at the end closest to you, make even folds that are approximately 1in/2cm wide, turning the paper over each time for a pleated effect. Press each fold flat (or use a ruler to rub over the fold to make it as flat as possible).

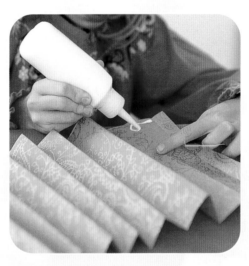

3 DECORATE To decorate the fan, open out the pleats slightly and use glue to create a swirling pattern along the top edge of the paper. Scatter glitter over the glue and shake to remove the excess. Allow the glue to dry before folding up the fan again.

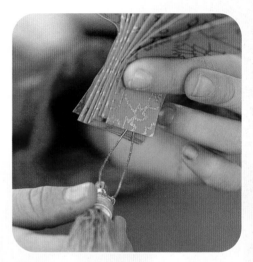

4 FINISHING Pinch the pleats at the bottom of the fan together, and insert the end of the silk tassel in between the central pleats. Use a stapler to secure the pleats (two or three staples are usually sufficient). If children are very young, an adult should be responsible for the stapling.

pressing flowers

The traditional art of flower pressing will delight young children and the finished items can be used to decorate all manner of objects. We used a flower press, but leaves and flowers can be easily pressed between the pages of a heavy book or telephone directory and left for a few days to dry out.

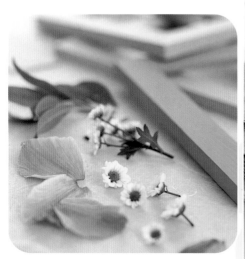

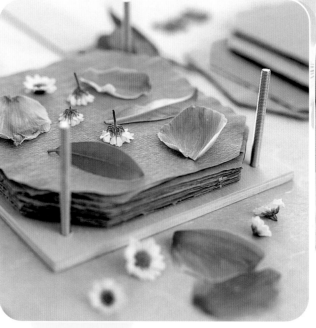

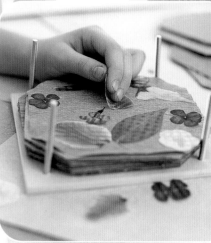

1 CHOOSE FLOWERS It is fun to pick the flowers from the garden, but if this is not possible use bought flowers. The flatter the flower, the easier it will be to press. If the flower is bulky, pull off the petals, press them individually and use them to recreate the flower once they are pressed.

2 PRESS FLOWERS Carefully place the flowers and leaves in the press between the layers of paper and card. Replace the top of the flower press and tighten the screws as firmly as you can. This ensures that as little air as possible can get to the flowers and leaves. An adult may need to help tighten the screws.

3 REMOVE FLOWERS The flowers and leaves should be left for about a week to make sure they are completely dry. Once they are dry, peel them away from the papers in the press as carefully as possible, since they become very fragile once they are dry. Place them on a sheet of paper ready for application.

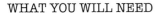

WHAT YOU WILL NEED

- ✿ flowers and leaves
- ✿ flower press
- ✿ object for decoration (e.g. bookmark, picture frame, or greetings card)
- ✿ glue
- ✿ brushes for glue
- ✿ tweezers for lifting flowers, if required

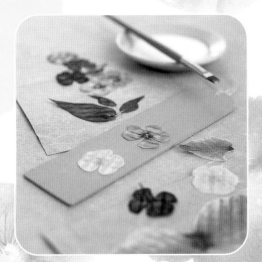

4 APPLY TO DESIRED OBJECT

Apply a thin layer of glue to the back of a flower. Gently lift the flower and place it in the required position (use tweezers if necessary). Add other flowers until the design is complete. Allow to dry thoroughly. If decorating a box, apply a layer of water-based acrylic varnish.

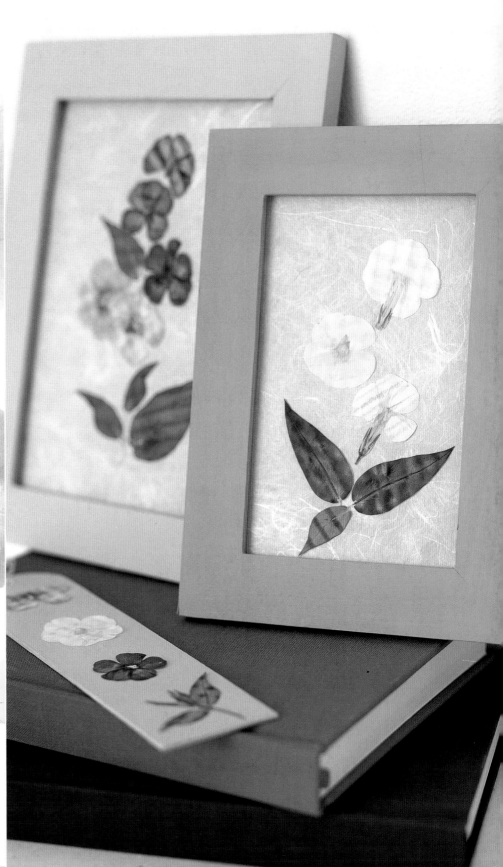

painted stones

Painted stones can be used to create a variety of items, such as paperweights, jewelry, and bookends. The shape of the stone may inspire its design—what does the stone look like, and what could it be made into?

WHAT YOU WILL NEED

✪ paint in your chosen colors
✪ paintbrushes in various sizes
✪ saucers to hold the paint
✪ one large stone for the body
✪ two small round stones for the eyes
✪ two flat oval-shaped stones for the feet
✪ strong glue

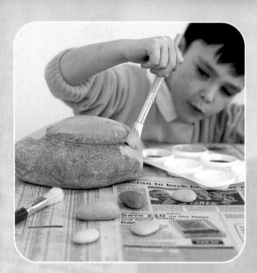

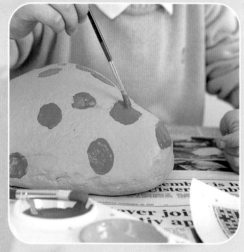

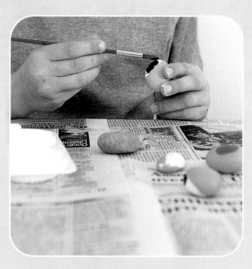

1 PAINT STONES Paint the large stone for the body green all over and allow to dry. For the best results, apply a second coat and let dry. We painted the top of the stone first, then the underside when the top was completely dry. Paint the smaller stones green, and let dry.

2 ADD THE DETAILS Paint on the spots using a darker shade of green paint. If you want very regular spots, draw them on the stone first, using a pencil. Fill in the spots using a finer paintbrush. Now use a very fine paintbrush and some white paint to paint on the frog's smiling mouth.

3 PAINT EYES AND FEET Paint the small round stones for the eyes with a circle of white paint for the frog's eyes, then leave to dry. Now, using a finer paintbrush, paint on the black eyeballs. Decorate the flatter oval stones for the frog's feet with dark green spots to match the body.

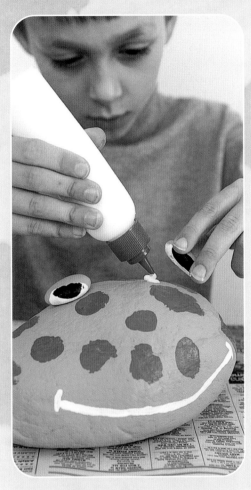

4 FINISHING Use strong glue to fix the frog's eyes to the top of the body. Repeat for the feet on the underside of the stone. Allow to dry completely.

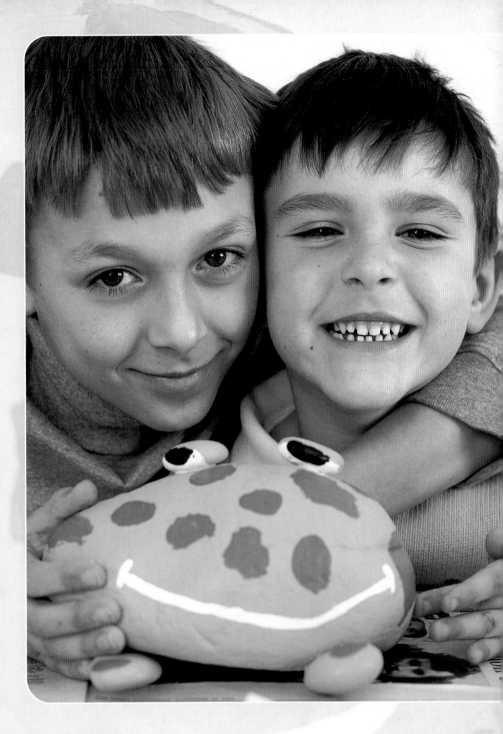

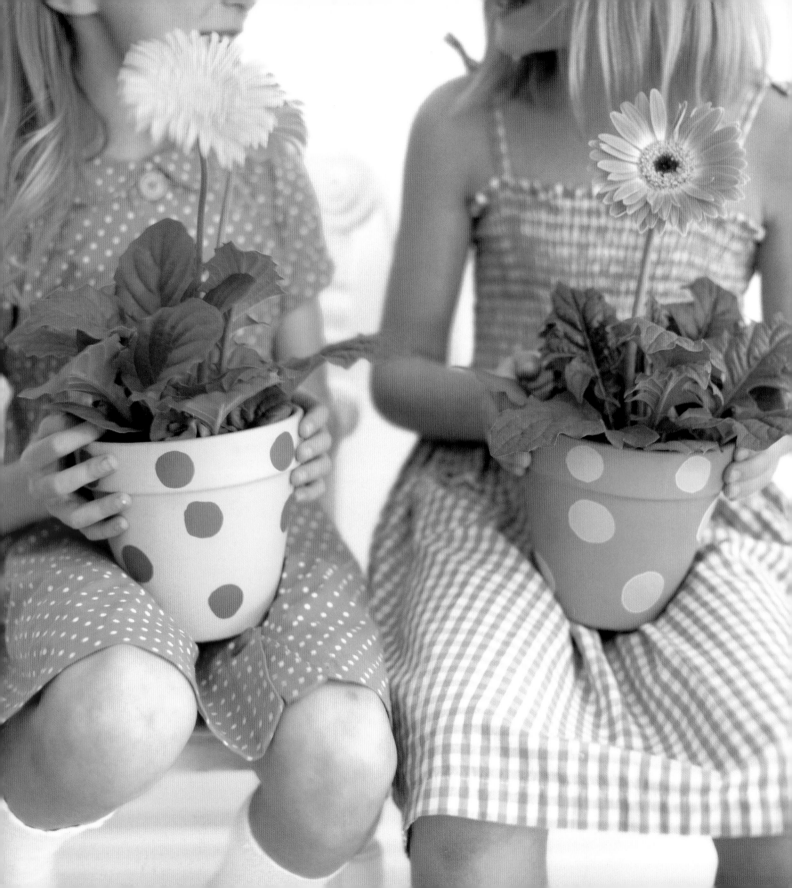

painted pots

These terracotta plant pots have been painted in fun bright shades then decorated with bold contrasting spots. Plant them up with cheerful annuals and display them indoors or out, or give them as gifts to friends and relatives.

WHAT YOU WILL NEED
✪ terracotta plant pots
✪ saucer for paint
✪ assorted paintbrushes
✪ undercoat
✪ colored paint
✪ pencil
✪ water-based acrylic varnish

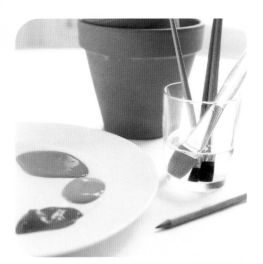

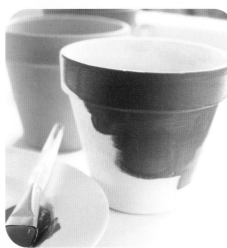

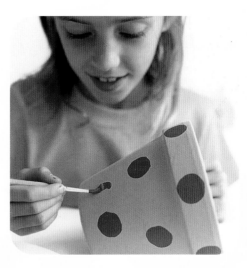

1 CHOOSE MATERIALS Apply undercoat to the pots and allow them to dry thoroughly. Paint the inside of the pot with the undercoat to about halfway down, so that the terracotta does not show. Apply a further coat if required.

2 PAINT BASE COLOR Now apply a coat of the base color to the outside and inside of the pot, and allow it to dry completely. For more even coverage, apply a further coat of paint and allow to dry.

3 FINISHING Use a pencil to carefully draw the spots on the outside of the pot. Apply the contrasting paint, using a fine brush to fill in the spots, and allow to dry. Finish the pot with a coat of hard-wearing water-based acrylic varnish.

modeling with balsa wood

Lightweight balsa wood is easy to cut and glue, which makes it ideal for children to use for modeling. Small pieces can be cut with scissors, but thicker pieces of balsa should be cut by an adult using a junior hacksaw.

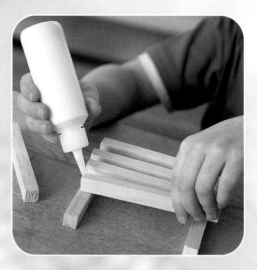

1 GLUE BASE Cut seven lengths of balsa wood measuring 4 x ½ x ½in/10 x 1 x 1cm for the base of the boat. Lay two pieces of the wood about 3½in/9cm apart and glue the other five pieces on the top at equal intervals. For the mast, cut two squares of wood measuring ½ x ½in/1 x 1cm and two lengths of 4 x ¼in/10cm x 5mm.

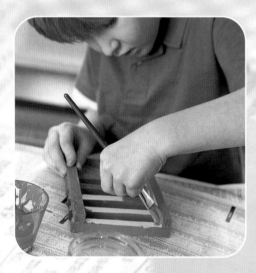

2 PAINT BASE Now paint the base of the boat and the mast sections and allow them to dry completely. You may need to apply a further coat of paint to ensure even coverage. Allow the paint to dry completely before attaching the mast.

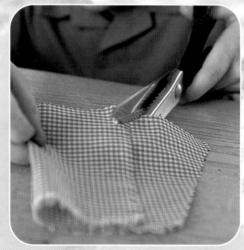

3 MAKE SAIL AND MAST Cut out a triangle of fabric 3 x 3in/8 x 8cm wide, using pinking shears to prevent the fabric from fraying. Lay one mast piece on the table and apply glue down the center of the fabric triangle before placing it on top. Lay the second mast on top, so the sail is sandwiched between the pieces of wood, then glue in place. Allow to dry.

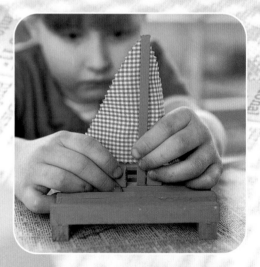

4 ATTACH SAIL Glue the base of the mast to the two squares of balsa wood so that it is held between them. Apply a blob of glue to the center of the boat base, and stick the sail and mast to the base. Allow the glue to dry. You may wish to apply more paint to cover the glue in this area.

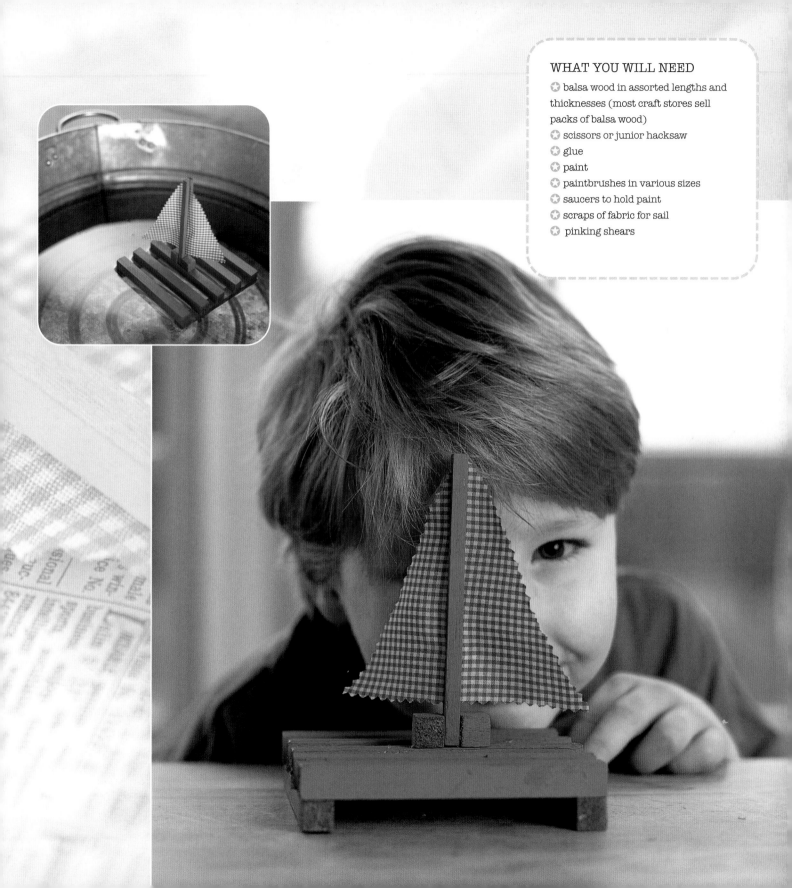

herb planter

Growing herbs is a great way to learn about edible plants, and they're a doddle to grow in a window box on a sunny window ledge or patio. For a never-ending supply of tasty leaves, all you need to do is keep on picking them!

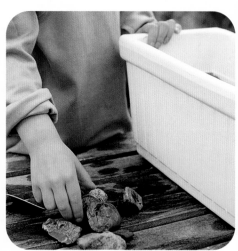

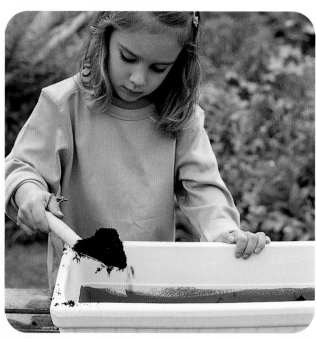

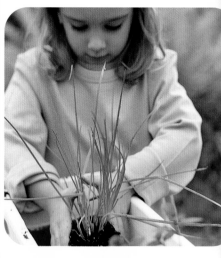

1 COVER HOLES Before filling your window box with compost, cover the drainage holes in the base. Use large stones or pieces of broken terracotta pot. This will allow water to drain away, but prevent the holes from getting clogged with compost. It will also prevent compost spilling through the holes and onto surfaces.

2 ADD COMPOST Cover the base of the container with a ½in/1cm-deep layer of potting mix, breaking any large clods apart with your hands. Roughly level the soil with your fingers to leave a smooth finish.

3 ARRANGE PLANTS Take your plants out of their containers and arrange them in the window box. Upright plants will look better in the center of the container, while creeping plants are best tumbling over the ends. Once you are happy with your display, fill the gaps around the plants with soil, leaving a level surface about 1in/2cm below the top of the trough. Firm around the plants with your fingertips and water them well.

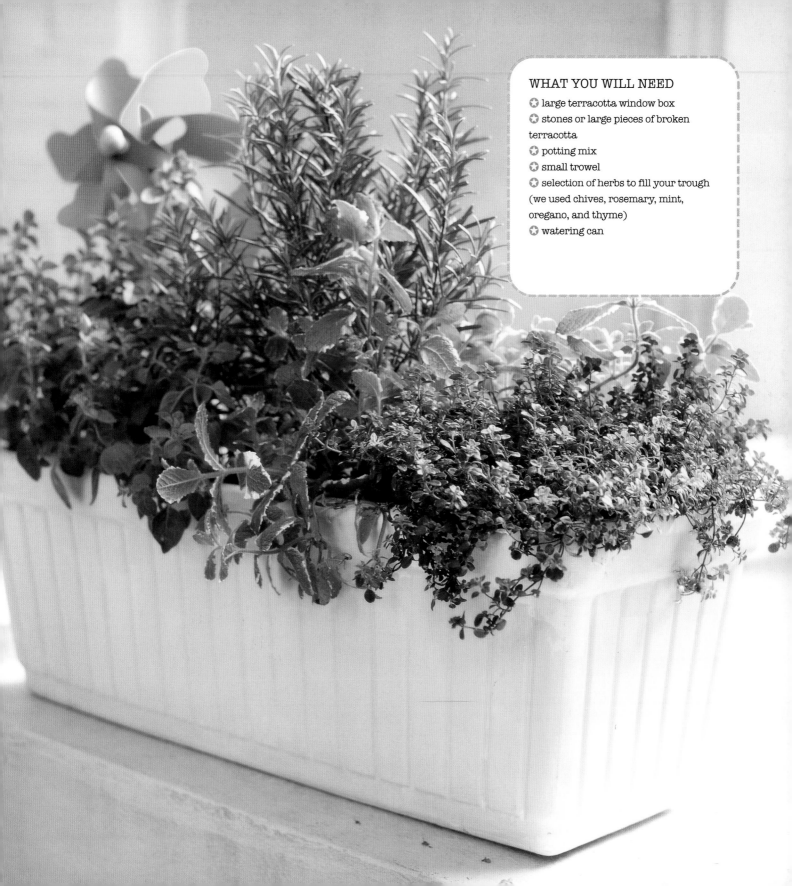

WHAT YOU WILL NEED

✪ large terracotta window box
✪ stones or large pieces of broken terracotta
✪ potting mix
✪ small trowel
✪ selection of herbs to fill your trough (we used chives, rosemary, mint, oregano, and thyme)
✪ watering can

harvesting herbs

During late spring and summer, herbs make lots of fresh new growth, which is perfect for harvesting and drying. Store dried herbs in cellophane bags, and keep them handy in the kitchen. They also make great presents to give to friends.

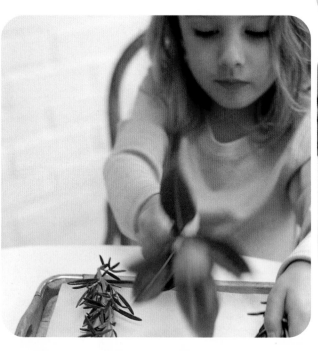

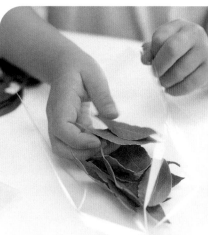

1 CUT HERBS Select a handful of fresh, healthy new shoots and snip them off with a pair of scissors. To ensure the parent plant is left in good shape, cut just above a pair of leaves. Fill a bowl with cold water and quickly dip the shoots to remove any dirt, then gently dry them on paper towels.

2 PREPARE TO DRY Cover a tray with a sheet of waxed paper and lay the shoots on top to dry. If you are drying different kinds of herbs, make sure they are not touching. Now put the tray in a warm, dark place until the herbs have dried completely.

3 FINISHING Carefully remove the individual leaves and put them into small cellophane bags. Fold over and secure the top of the bag to keep the contents fresh. Add a label, then store the herbs in a kitchen cupboard.

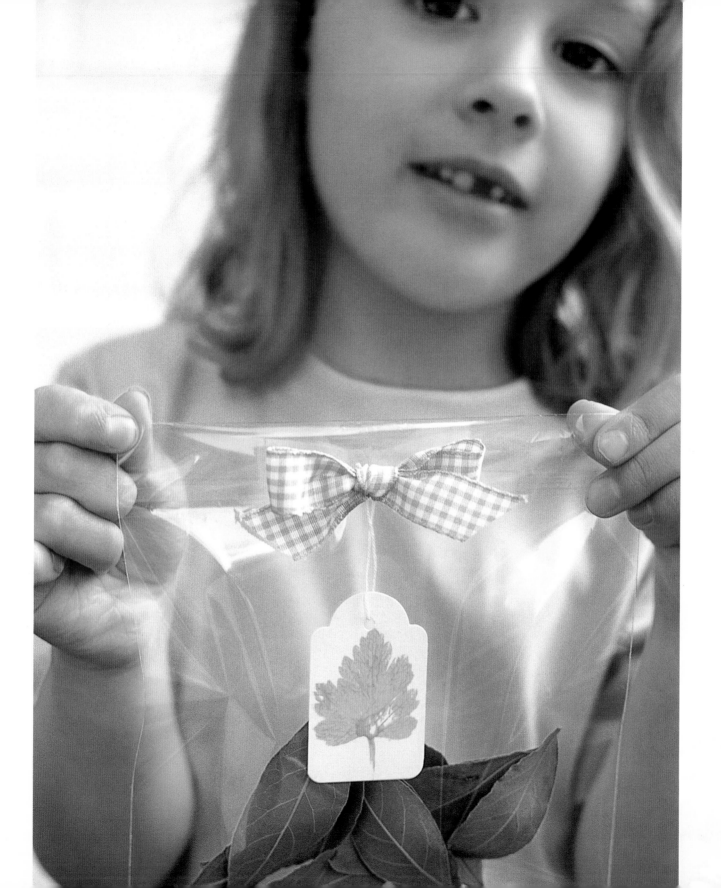

tie-dye t-shirt

Tie-dyeing is a simple process with striking results. You can give old white T-shirts a new lease on life with this technique, but it is is advisable to have an adult on hand, as it can get quite messy. Alternatively, follow the steps shown here to create the design, but use machine dye rather than the bucket method, as it's an easier (and less messy) option.

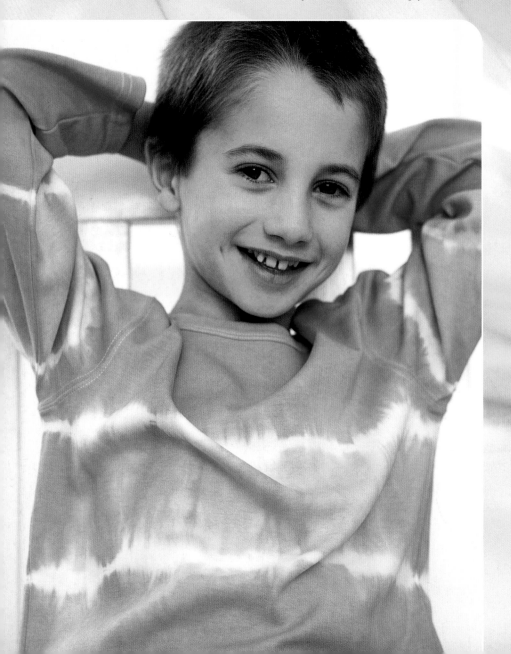

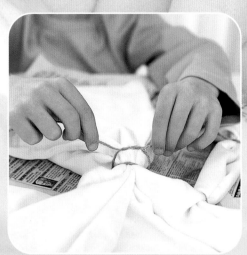

1 TIE UP MATERIAL Tie the string around the sleeves of the T-shirt in two places and pull tightly to ensure no dye can get through. Repeat on the body of the T-shirt, tying two pieces of string at 4in/10cm intervals. If you want additional stripes, tie more lengths of string around the T-shirt.

WHAT YOU WILL NEED

- ✿ T-shirt
- ✿ string
- ✿ dye in the color of your choice
- ✿ bucket
- ✿ jug
- ✿ wooden spoon
- ✿ scissors

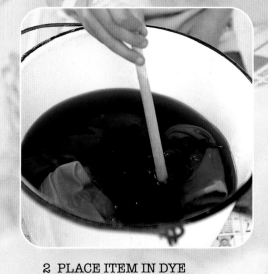

2 PLACE ITEM IN DYE
Following the manufacturer's instructions, make up the dye in a bucket, adding dye fix if necessary. Push the T-shirt into the bucket of dye and stir gently with a wooden spoon to ensure the fabric is evenly covered with the dye. Leave the T-shirt for approximately one hour, stirring occasionally.

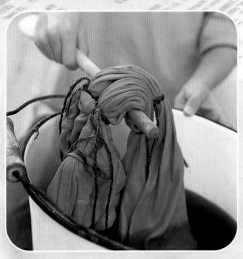

3 REMOVE THE T-SHIRT When the dye process is complete, carefully remove the T-shirt from the bucket and wash the items according to the dye manufacturer's instructions. Leave the strings in place on the T-shirt.

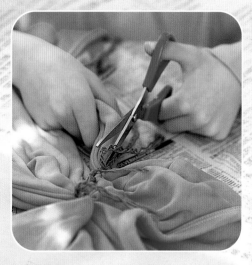

4 CUT THE STRINGS Allow the T-shirt to dry completely. Now use a pair of scissors to carefully cut the strings, taking care not to damage the T-shirt. Ask an adult to help iron the T-shirt to remove the crease marks left by the string.

crystallized pansies

Real pansies make the daintiest of decorations for a plate of cute cupcakes, and they even taste good too! Egg white and superfine sugar is all that you need to create these pretty crystallized flowers.

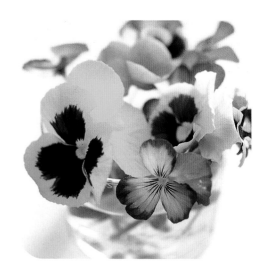

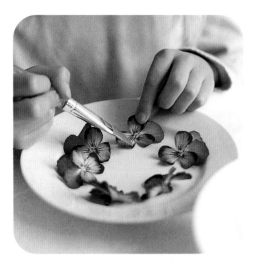

1 PAINT ON EGG WHITE
Using a fine paintbrush, paint each flower with egg white. Paint no more than five or six flowers at a time, as the egg white tends to dry quite quickly.

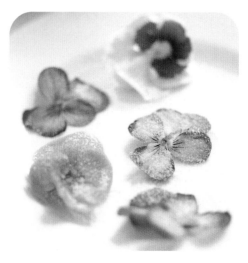

2 SPRINKLE ON SUGAR Use a spoon to gently sprinkle the sugar over the flowers, making sure not to add too much. Leave to dry. The flowers will become hard and brittle.

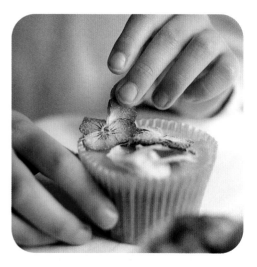

3 FINISHING Use two or three of the crystallized flowers to decorate each cupcake. Serve on a pretty cake plate or glass cakestand.

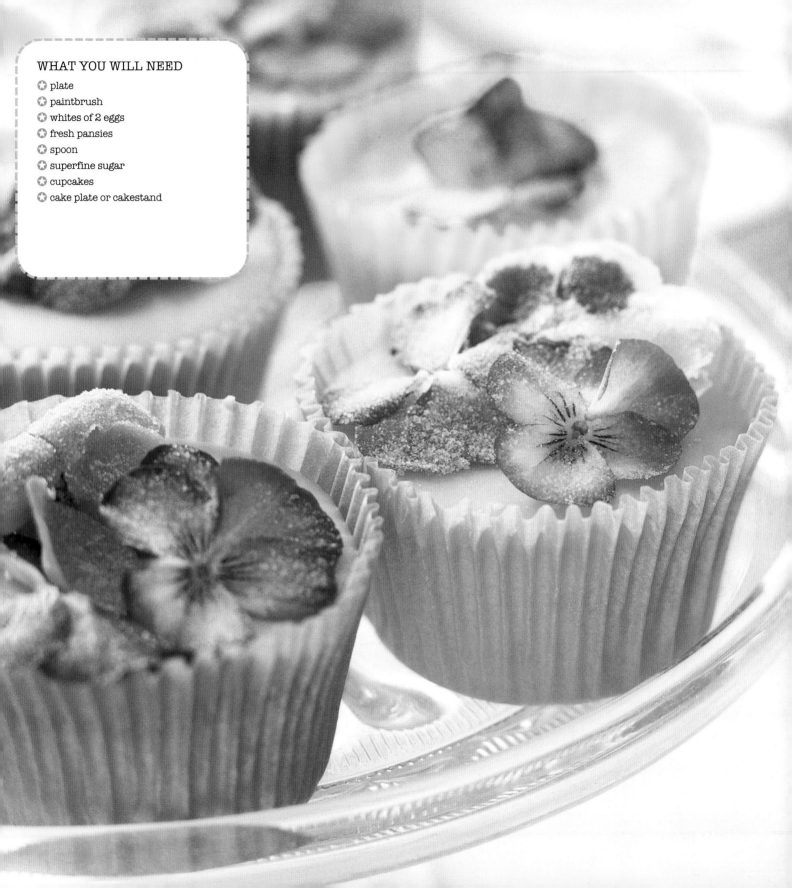

WHAT YOU WILL NEED

- ✪ plate
- ✪ paintbrush
- ✪ whites of 2 eggs
- ✪ fresh pansies
- ✪ spoon
- ✪ superfine sugar
- ✪ cupcakes
- ✪ cake plate or cakestand

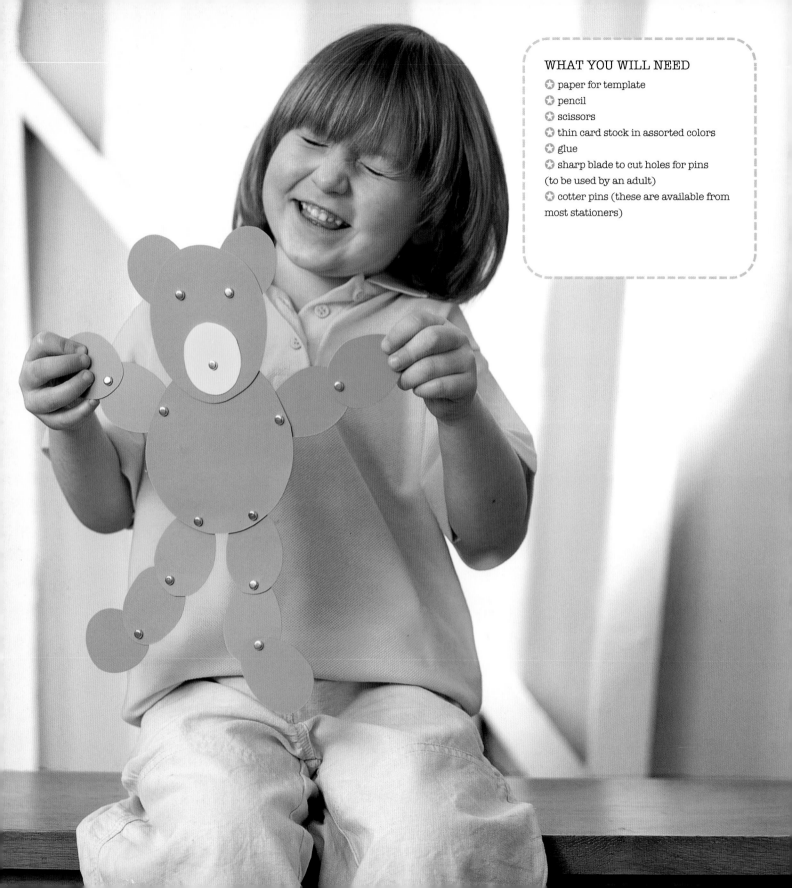

WHAT YOU WILL NEED

✪ paper for template
✪ pencil
✪ scissors
✪ thin card stock in assorted colors
✪ glue
✪ sharp blade to cut holes for pins
(to be used by an adult)
✪ cotter pins (these are available from
most stationers)

cotter-pin animals

Cotter-pin animals are fun to make and educational, too, as they teach young children about joints and movement. As you cut out and make the animals, describe how the sections will move when held together by the cotter pins. They can also be used decoratively, to make buttons and eyes for the creatures.

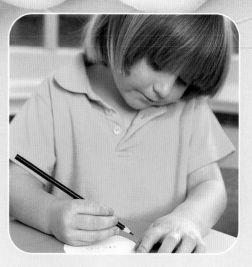

1 CUT OUT Trace the teddy templates on page 153 onto plain paper and cut them out. Draw around the templates on a piece of card stock and cut them out. You will need twelve identical-sized ovals for the teddy's legs, arms and ears, then one each for the nose, head and body. We used different-colored card for the teddy's nose.

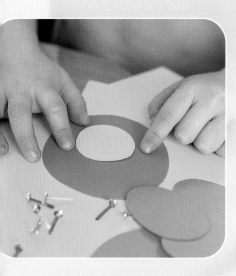

2 GLUE ON NOSE Use glue to stick the nose to the teddy's face and allow it to dry completely. Lay out all the pieces of the teddy bear on a table so you can work out where the positions for the holes should be.

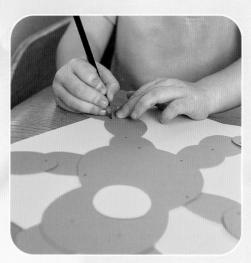

3 MARK AND CUT HOLES Use a pencil to mark the holes for the pins, making sure that each of the card sections overlap at this point, so they will be held together by the pins. Use a sharp blade to make slits through the layers of card. It is advisable for an adult to do this, as sharp blades are dangerous.

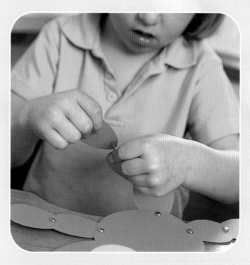

4 INSERT THE PINS Insert the cotter pins through each slit and fold them flat at the back of the bear. Continue until the whole teddy has been assembled. We added a decorative pin through the teddy's nose as a finishing touch.

colorful annuals

Annuals will fill your garden with cheerful color. Buy them as plants in early summer and they will flower non-stop through until autumn. For a really fun, jazzy display, use your imagination and plant them in the most unusual containers you can find.

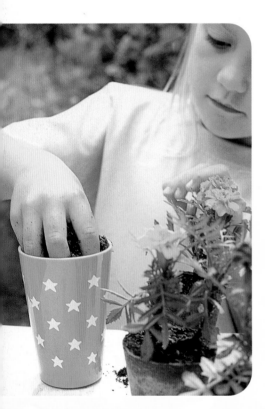

1 ADD SOIL Put a handful of potting mix in the bottom of a beaker. Don't worry about drainage holes, as annual plants only last for a short time.

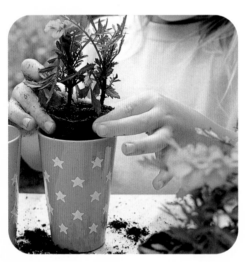

2 PLANT UP Sit a plant on top of the potting mix. The surface of the rootball needs to be just beneath the lip of the pot, so add or remove soil as necessary.

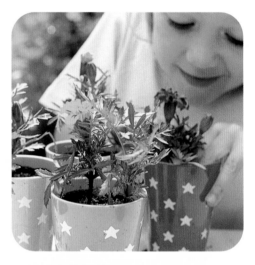

3 FINISHING Use more potting mix to fill any gaps around the edges of the rootball and firm down with your fingertips. Water the plants, but don't overdo it, as the beaker doesn't have any drainage holes. Add some water, allow it to soak in, then test by pushing your finger into the soil. If it's thoroughly wet, you don't need to add any more.

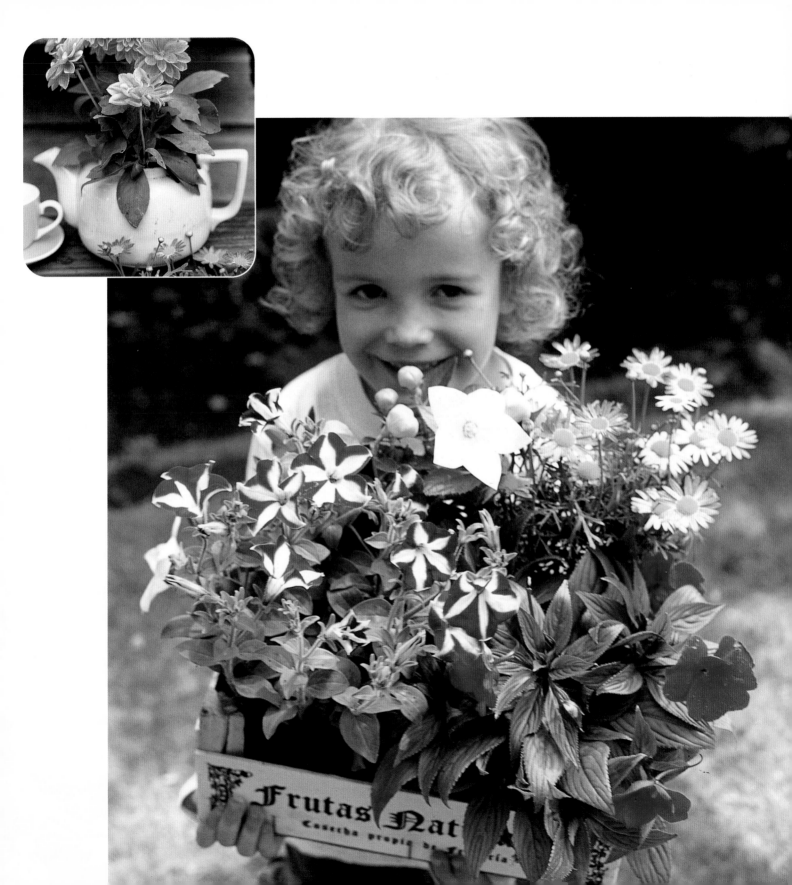

father's day gift

These decorative keyrings are made from balsa wood and thin wood sheets, and make the perfect gift for Father's Day. Key chains are available from craft stores and are easily attached to the wood. Both boys and girls will enjoy this easy woodwork technique.

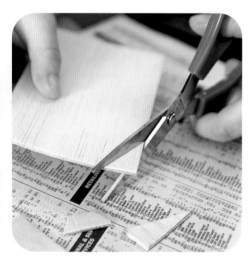

1 CUT SIMPLE SHAPES Cut small rectangles from the wood sheet. This will be the base of the keyring. Now draw simple motifs straight onto the balsa wood and cut them out using scissors. An adult may need to assist a younger child in cutting the wood.

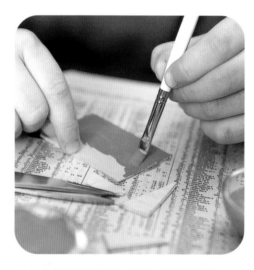

2 PAINT BASE AND CUTOUTS Paint the base of the keyring all over the back and front and allow to dry. A further coat of paint may be necessary for even coverage. Paint the front and edges of the smaller balsa-wood pieces using a fine paintbrush. Allow to dry.

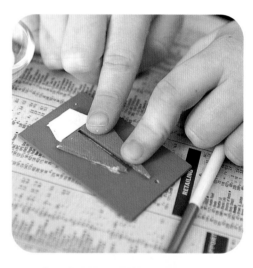

3 GLUE ON MOTIF Apply glue to the back of the balsa-wood pieces and stick them in place on the front of the keyring. Press down firmly. Allow the glue to dry completely. You may wish to apply a coat of water-based acrylic varnish to make the keyring more hard-wearing.

WHAT YOU WILL NEED

- ✪ thin wood sheet (available from craft stores)
- ✪ scissors
- ✪ balsa wood
- ✪ pencil
- ✪ paint in your chosen colors
- ✪ saucer to hold paints
- ✪ paintbrushes in various sizes
- ✪ glue
- ✪ awl
- ✪ keyring attachment

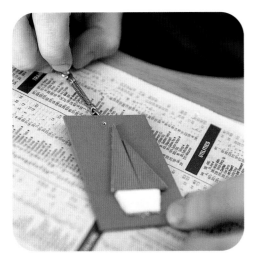

4 ATTACH CHAIN Make a small hole at the top of the keyring using an awl. For safety reasons, it is advisable for an adult to do this part of the project. Take the keyring attachment, thread the metal loop through the hole, and close using pliers.

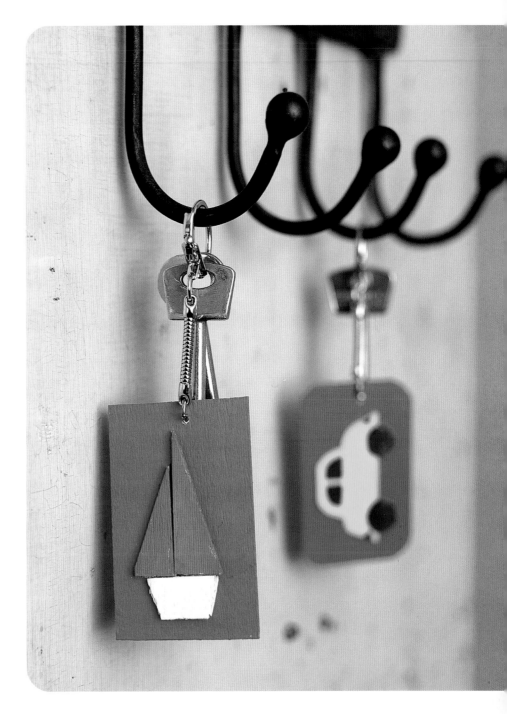

pretty plant labels

Jumbo craft sticks with butterfly-shaped ends make pretty plant markers that identify plants growing in pots or the garden. Paint them in strong pastel shades that will stand out against the lush green of foliage, and write the name of the plant on in pencil.

WHAT YOU WILL NEED
- paint
- small paintbrushes
- natural wood jumbo craft sticks
- undercoat
- pencil

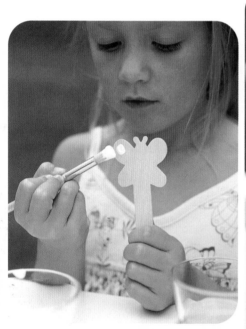

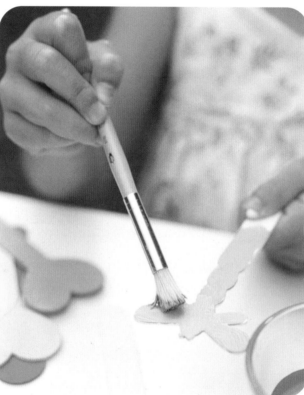

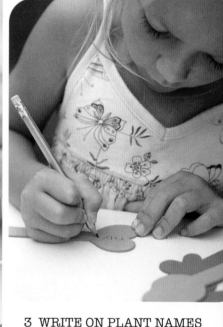

1 APPLY UNDERCOAT
Use a small paintbrush to apply a coat of undercoat to the craft stick. Let it dry completely and add a second coat if the coverage is patchy.

2 PAINT MARKERS
When the undercoat is completely dry, apply paint in your chosen color to one side and the edges of a craft stick, and leave it to dry. Next, paint the other side of the stick and, again, leave it to dry. Apply a further coat, if required.

3 WRITE ON PLANT NAMES
Once the painted markers are completely dry, write on the plant names. There is usually a tag or sticky label on the pot that a plant comes in (or on a seed packet, if you have grown it from seed). Copy this in clear, bold writing. Now the marker is ready to be pushed into the earth alongside the plant that it identifies.

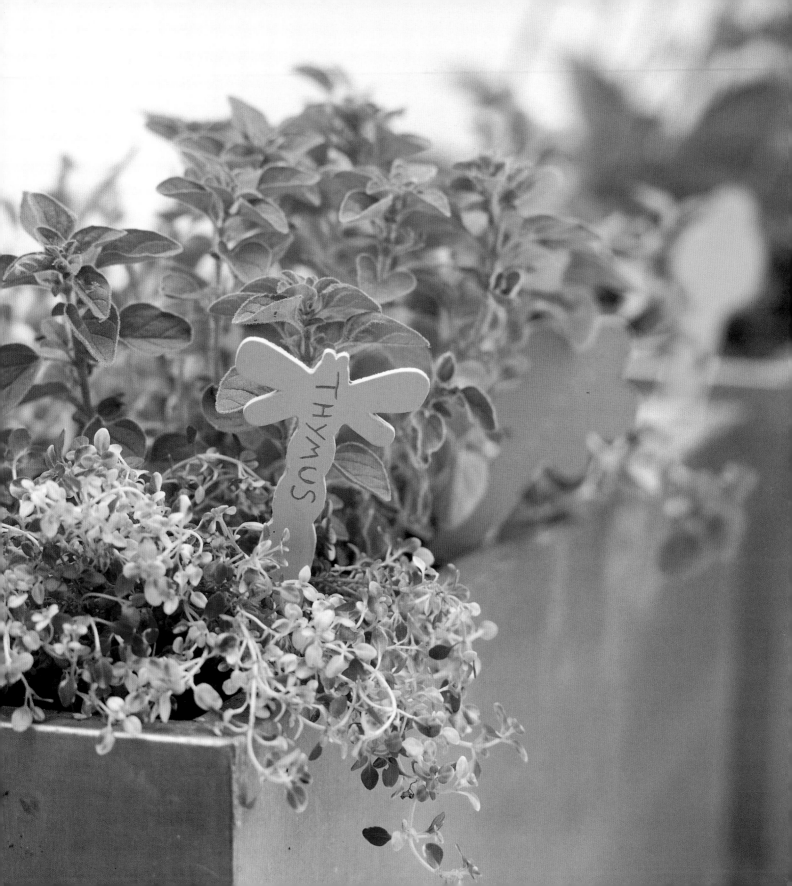

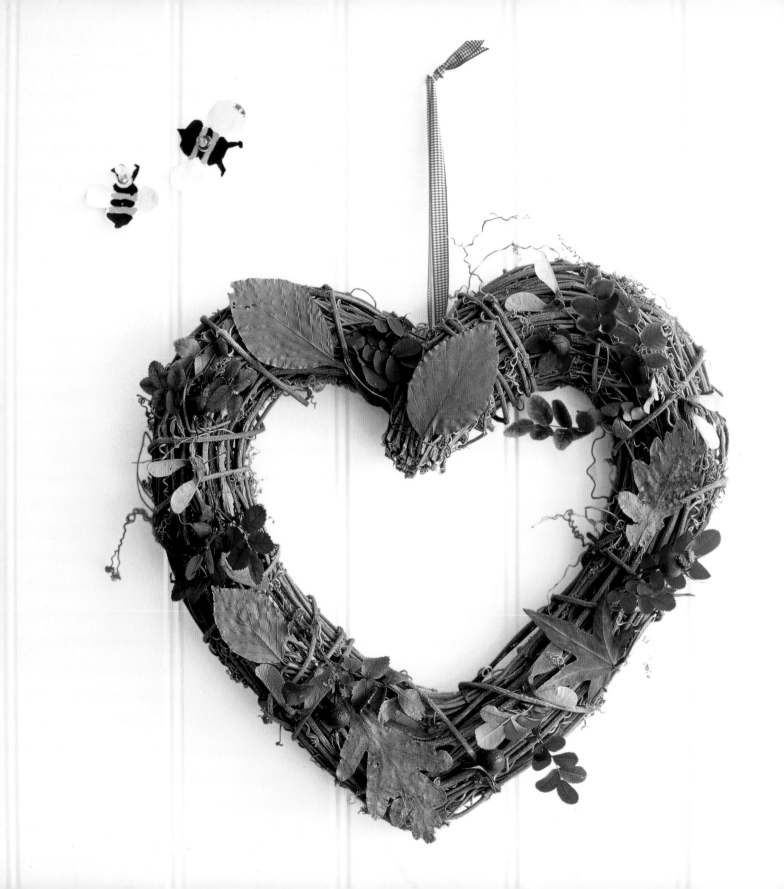

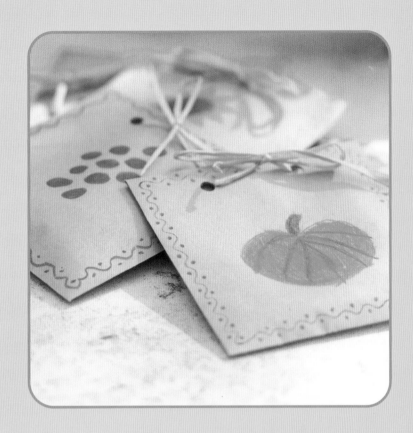

fall

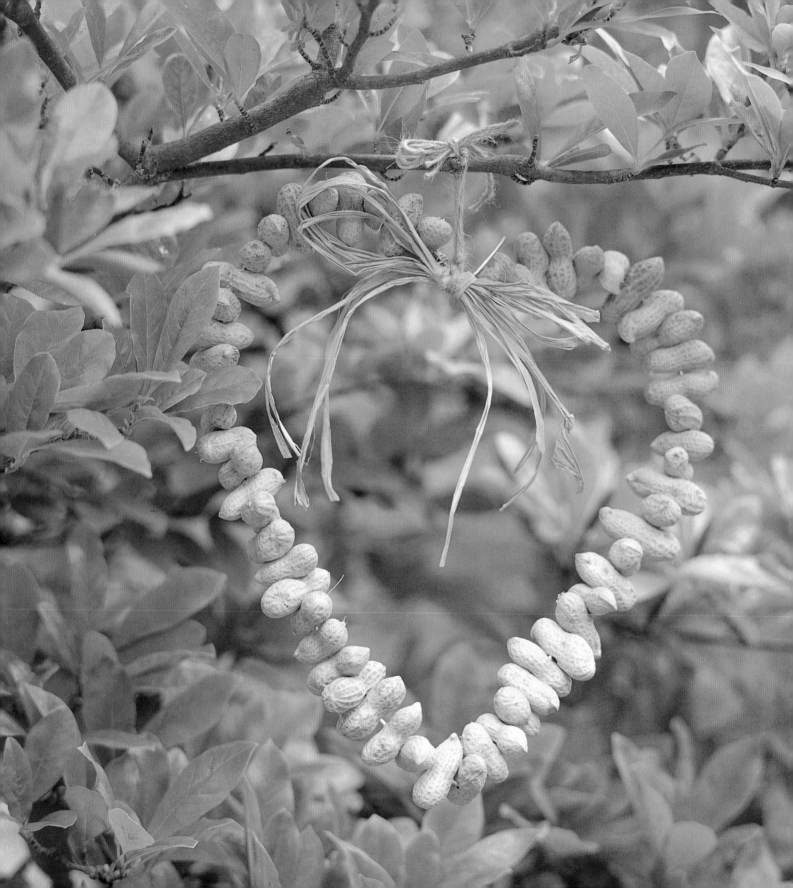

peanut heart

Unshelled peanuts can be easily pierced and threaded onto wire to create a bird feeder that our feathered friends will appreciate during the winter months. We finished off this heart-shaped feeder with a raffia bow to create a pretty and practical garden ornament.

WHAT YOU WILL NEED
- ✪ unshelled peanuts
- ✪ wooden skewer or awl for piercing holes
- ✪ strong wire
- ✪ raffia for bow
- ✪ 8in/20cm twine for hanging loop

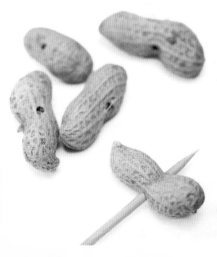

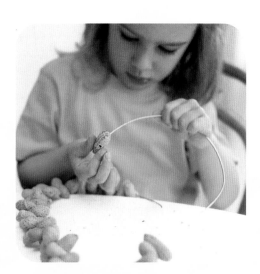

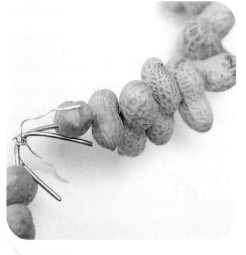

1 PIERCE HOLES IN PEANUTS
Ask an adult to pierce the holes in the nuts using a wooden skewer or an awl. You will need approximately 60 peanuts to make one peanut heart.

2 THREAD PEANUTS
Fold the wire in half to create the "V" shape of the heart. Begin threading peanuts onto the wire. Each side needs around 30 peanuts.

3 FINISHING
Ask an adult to bend each side of the heart into a curve to form a heart shape and to twist the wire to fix the ends in place. Now tie a raffia bow at the top of the heart to cover the wire ends. Cut an 8in/20cm length of twine to form the hanging loop, and suspend your bird feeder from a tree branch.

covering books

Use pretty handmade paper to cover textbooks or notebooks. You can use them at school or give them as gifts. The same technique can be used to decorate boxes or photograph albums, which make welcome keepsakes.

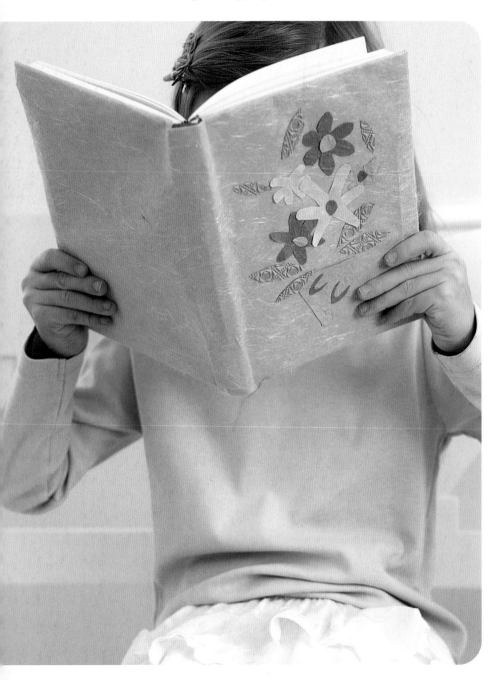

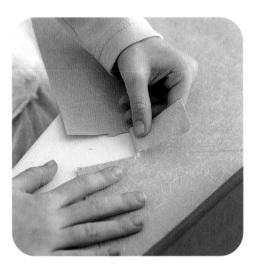

1 CUT OUT PAPER Lay the book flat on the piece of decorative paper. Cut all around the book, leaving a margin of about 1 ¹⁄₂in/4cm paper around the sides. Where the spine of the book lies, cut two slits in the paper at the top and bottom of the book, and neatly fold them inwards to hide them.

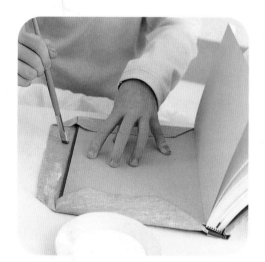

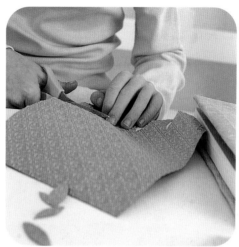

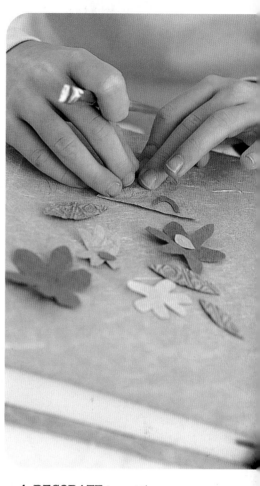

3 CUT OUT DECORATIONS Use scissors to cut out flowers, petals, and whatever other decorations are desired. These can be drawn using a pencil first, or cut out freehand, depending on the child.

2 GLUE ON COVER Fold the remaining edges of the paper towards the inside of the book and make pleated folds at the corners to neaten the edges. Glue the paper in place and allow to dry completely. It is a good idea to glue each layer of paper at the folded corners so they stay in place.

4 DECORATE Lay out the paper shapes on the book to create the design. When you are happy with your arrangement, glue each piece in place. If the pieces are small, use a fine paintbrush to apply the glue to the back of the paper. Allow to dry thoroughly.

indoor garden

You don't need to have a garden to grow plants. Small houseplants can be planted together in large glass jars to create an eye-catching display that needs very little watering or care. These gardens in a bottle look great when placed on a windowsill or shelf.

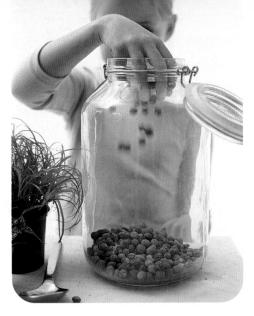

1 ADD CLAY PELLETS Make sure the inside of the glass container is clean (so you can see the plants!) then slowly pour in your clay pellets to make a 2in/5cm drainage layer in the base of the jar.

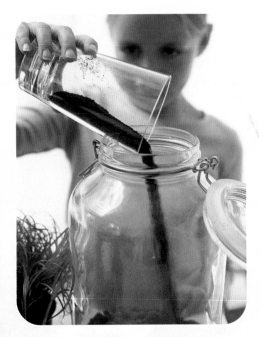

2 POUR IN CHARCOAL
Permanently damp soil can become smelly, so pour a thin layer of horticultural charcoal over the clay pellets, to keep it fresh.

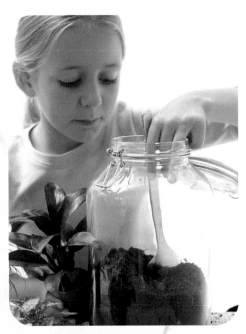

3 FILL WITH COMPOST Fill a quarter of the container with soil and press it down with your fingers (if your wrist can't fit freely through the neck of the bottle, use the back of a long-handled spoon to press the soil down).

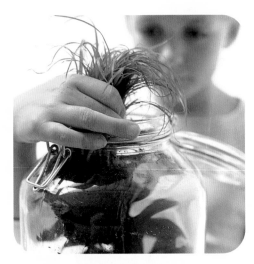

4 PLANT UP JAR Use the long-handled spoon to excavate small planting holes and lower plants into position. Firm the soil around the rootballs with the spoon. When you have finished planting, drop in some more clay pellets to cover any bare patches.

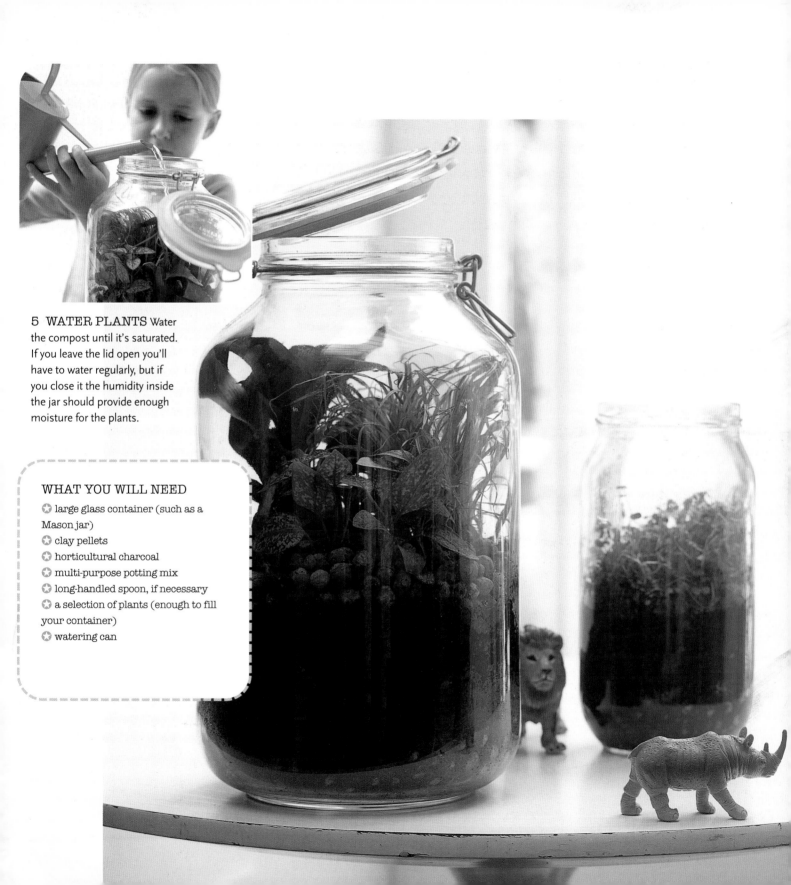

5 WATER PLANTS Water the compost until it's saturated. If you leave the lid open you'll have to water regularly, but if you close it the humidity inside the jar should provide enough moisture for the plants.

WHAT YOU WILL NEED

- ✪ large glass container (such as a Mason jar)
- ✪ clay pellets
- ✪ horticultural charcoal
- ✪ multi-purpose potting mix
- ✪ long-handled spoon, if necessary
- ✪ a selection of plants (enough to fill your container)
- ✪ watering can

finger puppets

Even younger children will enjoy making these animal finger puppets from felt. Very young children can glue rather than stitch them, as this eliminates the problem of sharp needles. Look through picture books for other ideas, and ask your child to draw any other animals he or she would like to make.

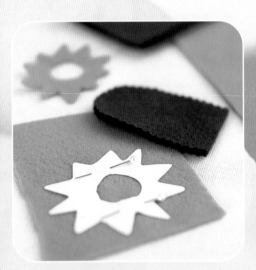

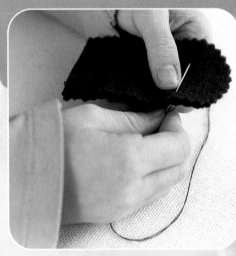

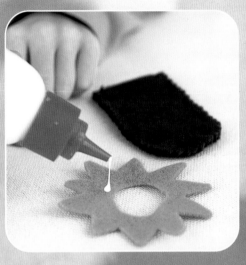

1 PIN AND CUT OUT Trace the templates on page 154 onto paper and cut them out. Pin the templates to the felt. Carefully cut out the felt. You will need two body shapes per puppet. We used pinking shears to cut out the bodies, but normal scissors will do, as felt does not fray.

2 SEW BODY PIECES TOGETHER Holding two body pieces together, hand-stitch around the edges using a running stitch in matching thread. Leave the bottom section open. If younger children are unable to sew, the edges can be glued together. When making the sheep puppet, fold a pleat in the base of the two ear shapes (as shown on the template) and tuck the ends of the ears inside the body sections before stitching in place.

3 GLUE ON THE HEADS For the lion puppet, apply neat dots of glue to the back of the mane and carefully place it on the front of the finger puppet. Push down firmly, then allow to dry completely. For the sheep puppet, glue on the little white face section and allow to dry.

WHAT YOU WILL NEED

- paper for templates
- pencil
- scissors
- pins
- squares of felt in assorted colors
- pinking shears
- needle and thread
- glue
- three-dimensional fabric paint

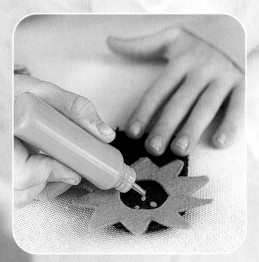

4 FINISHING Use three-dimensional fabric paint to carefully draw the nose and eyes onto the finger puppets. Allow to dry completely before starting to play.

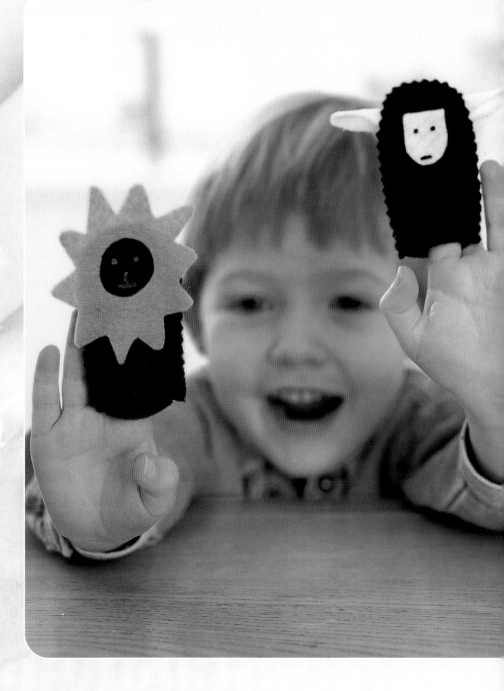

modeling with clay

Children love working with clay, and it can be used to create fun jewelry for friends, alphabet letters for doors, and funky fridge magnets. Cookie cutters come in all sorts of shapes and sizes, and cut clay easily. Once dry, your clay shapes can be colorfully painted and decorated.

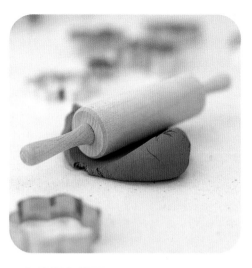

1 ROLL OUT Remove the clay from its packaging and knead to soften it. Roll the clay out with a rolling pin. For smaller objects such as brooches, the clay should be about ¼in/5mm thick. For larger items, the clay should be about ½in/1cm thick.

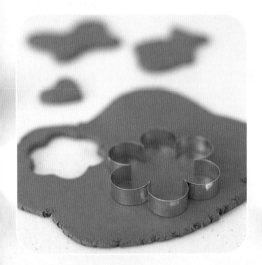

2 CUT OUT Use assorted cookie cutters to cut the shapes from the clay. Carefully remove the excess clay from around the cutter before removing it. If you are making a necklace, use a drinking straw to pierce a ribbon hole. Use a spatula to lift the clay shape and place on a tray to allow it to dry. When the top is dry, turn the shape over so the other side can dry completely.

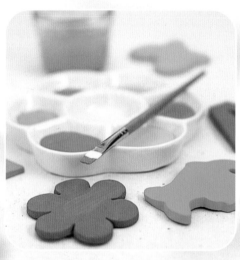

3 PAINT AND DECORATE Paint your clay shapes using brightly colored paints. You will probably need two or three layers of paint to achieve total coverage, but remember to allow each layer to dry thoroughly between coats. Paler colors will need more coats than darker shades.

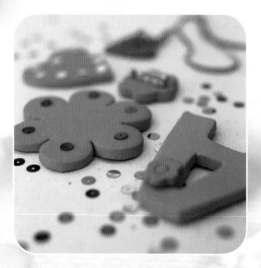

4 FINISHING Decorate the finished clay shapes with sequins or smaller clay shapes using a tiny dab of glue. You may need to use tweezers to position sequins on the shapes. Stick magnets to the back for fridge magnets, or use ribbon to make pendants. Use self-adhesive pads if you want to stick the letters to a door.

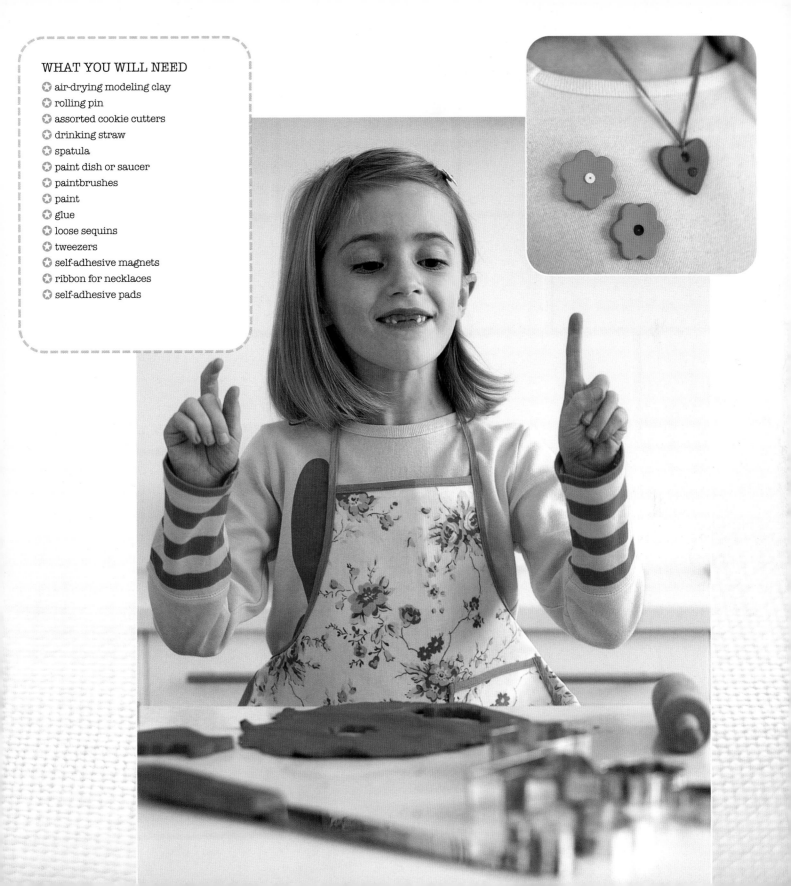

WHAT YOU WILL NEED

- air-drying modeling clay
- rolling pin
- assorted cookie cutters
- drinking straw
- spatula
- paint dish or saucer
- paintbrushes
- paint
- glue
- loose sequins
- tweezers
- self-adhesive magnets
- ribbon for necklaces
- self-adhesive pads

birdseed feeder

Attract wild birds to your garden with this fun birdseed feeder.
We made it from a pumpkin, which was then decorated with cloves
and filled with a generous heap of birdseed. Hang it from a tree in
your garden and watch the birds tuck in!

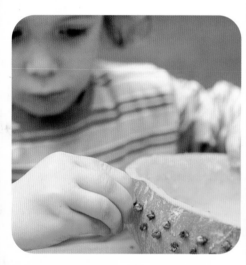

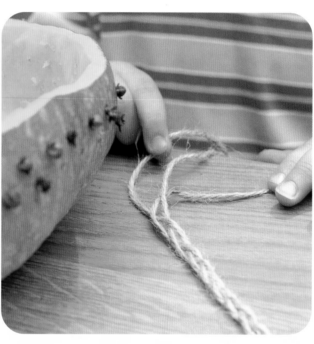

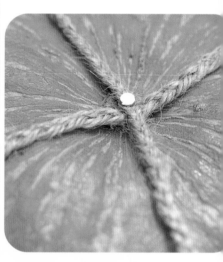

1 CUT PUMPKIN IN HALF
Ask an adult to cut the pumpkin in half
and scoop out the flesh from the inside
(the seeds can be used to make the
necklace on pages 98–99). The holes
for the cloves are pierced using an awl,
so it is advisable for an adult to do this.
Insert the cloves around the edge of
the squash in two parallel rows.

2 PLAIT STRING Cut six 3ft/1m-long
pieces of string. Take three strands and knot
them together at one end. Start plaiting the
string (it may be easier if someone helps you
by holding the knotted end). When the first
length is finished, plait the remaining three
lengths to form the second hanging loop.

3 FIX HANGING LOOPS Turn the
squash upside down. Lay the plaited string
in an 'X' across the base. Ask an adult to
push in a nail to hold the string in place.

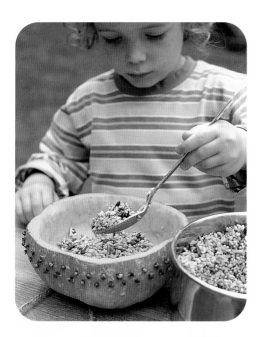

4 FINISHING Melt the packet of suet in a saucepan, until it becomes liquid. Add the birdseed and stir until the mix becomes firm. Carefully spoon the mixture into the pumpkin. Tie the ends of the string around a branch of a tree and, if necessary, trim the ends using scissors.

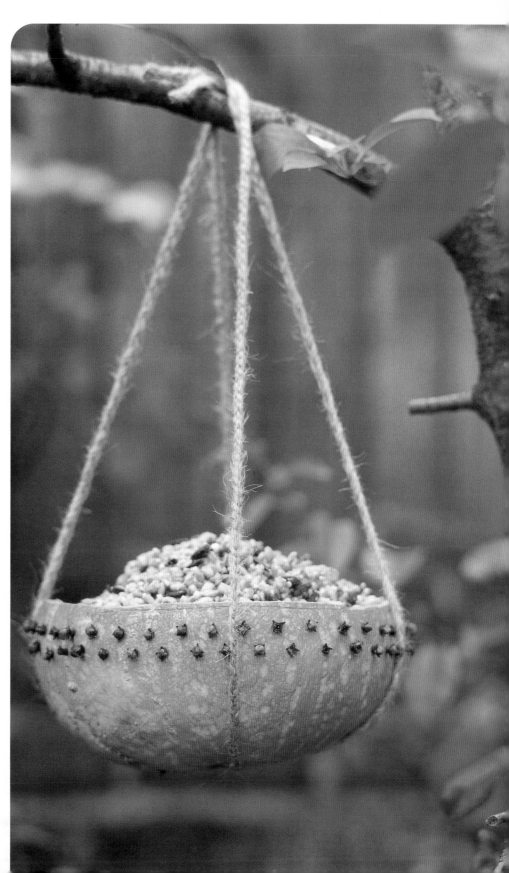

harvest wreath

Decorate a ready-made wreath with your own dried leaves to create a decorative harvest wreath to hang on the wall or front door. Collect a variety of attractive, different-colored leaves in autumn and use a flower press or large book to press them flat.

WHAT YOU WILL NEED
- dried leaves
- paper
- flower press or thick book
- heart-shaped wreath
- glue
- dried seedheads and sycamore wings
- 10in/25cm red gingham ribbon

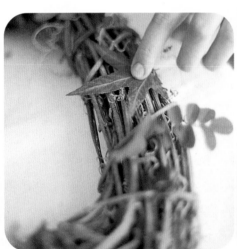

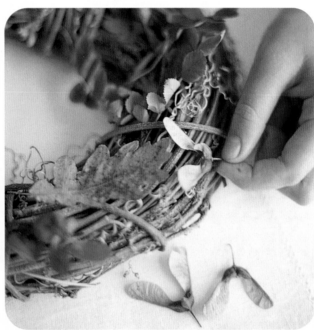

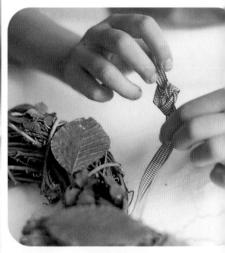

1 COLLECT AND DRY LEAVES Collect leaves for drying, making sure they are not damp. Place them between layers of paper in a thick book or flower press and leave for two or three weeks until dry. Put a dab of glue on the back of each leaf, and attach to the heart wreath.

2 GLUE ON LEAVES Continue to glue leaves to the wreath and add sycamore wings and dried seedheads at regular intervals. Allow the glue to dry completely.

3 FINISHING Thread the gingham ribbon through the top of the heart wreath. Knot the ends, and you will have a hanging loop that you can suspend the wreath from.

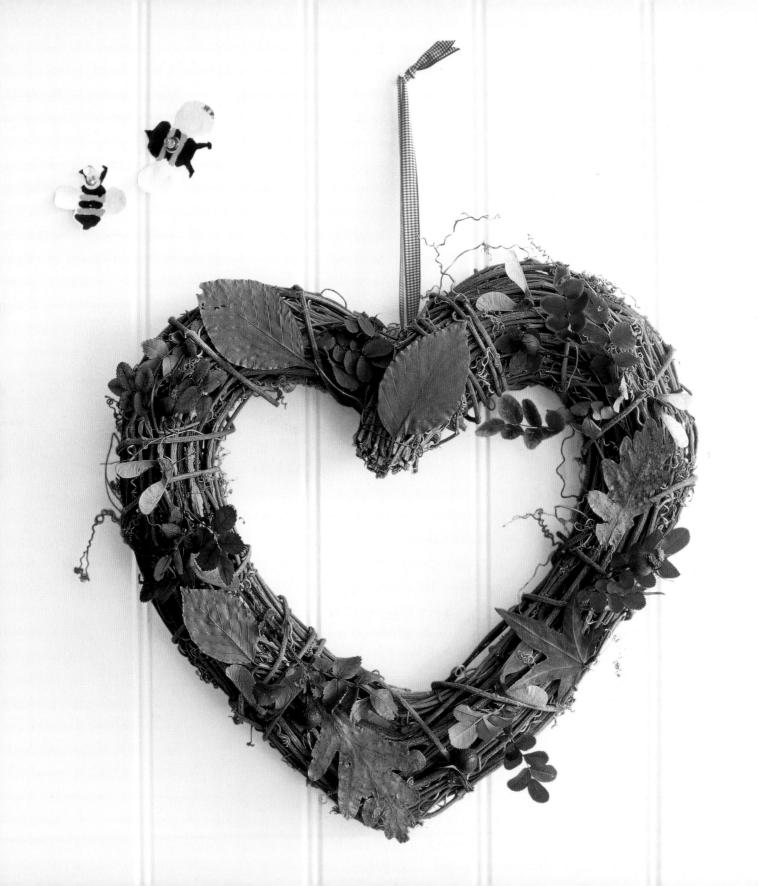

cat mask

This fun cat mask is perfect for Halloween or a dress-up party. Black is the best choice for Halloween, but it would look equally cute in brown or white. Add some pipe-cleaner whiskers and a little pompom for the cat's nose.

WHAT YOU WILL NEED
- ✪ tracing paper
- ✪ pencil
- ✪ scissors
- ✪ black card stock
- ✪ black felt
- ✪ glue
- ✪ pompom for nose
- ✪ pipe-cleaners for whiskers
- ✪ hole punch
- ✪ length of elastic

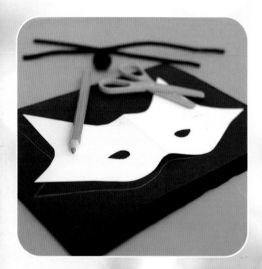

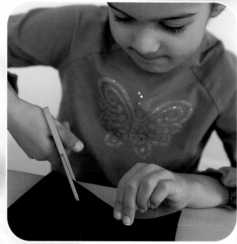

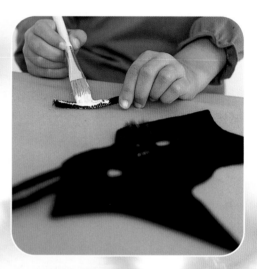

1 DRAW TEMPLATES Trace the mask template on page 154 onto a piece of folded card stock and cut it out. Open out the template. Take the piece of black felt and glue it to the piece of black card stock. Allow to dry.

2 CUT OUT MASK Draw around the paper template on the card side of the glued card and felt. Carefully cut out with scissors, taking particular care when cutting out the eye holes. An adult may need to help by first making a slit in the card for the eyes, so that the scissors can be easily inserted for cutting.

3 ATTACH NOSE AND WHISKERS Glue the pompom nose onto the mask. Cut six pipe-cleaner whiskers measuring approximately 4in/10cm in length, and glue them to each side of the mask, just below the eye holes. Allow to dry.

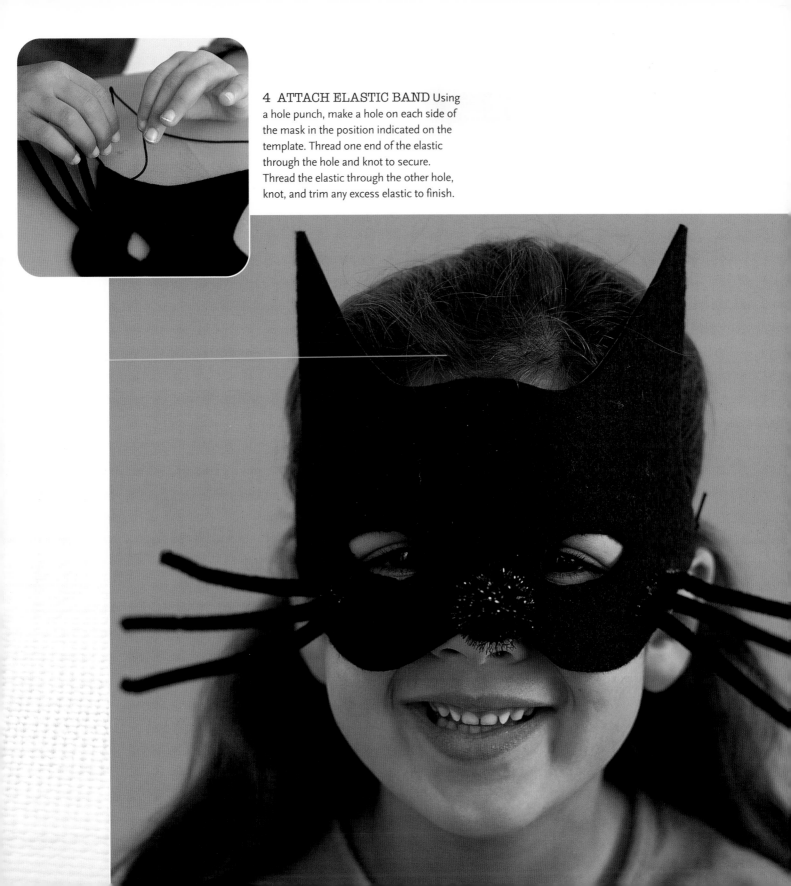

4 ATTACH ELASTIC BAND Using a hole punch, make a hole on each side of the mask in the position indicated on the template. Thread one end of the elastic through the hole and knot to secure. Thread the elastic through the other hole, knot, and trim any excess elastic to finish.

mirror-image painting

This is a perfect project for toddlers, who will be fascinated by the process. You may have to do the painting in stages—for example, the lion's face first, then the mane—otherwise the paint dries too quickly.

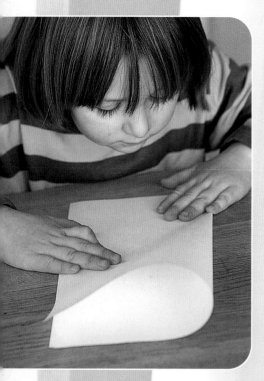

1 FOLD PAPER IN HALF Fold the paper in half, pressing down flat to form a crease. Open up the paper and draw a semicircle on one side of the paper in pencil (you may like to use a plate to draw a more accurate circle).

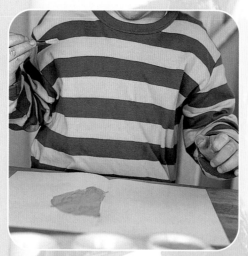

2 START PAINTING Fill in the semicircle with paint. It is important to do this fairly quickly, or the paint will start to dry and will not transfer properly to the other side of the paper when it is folded.

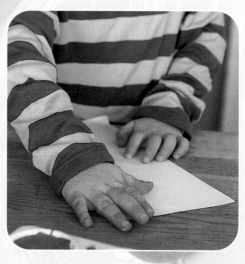

3 FOLD OVER Fold the paper in half on the original crease and press down firmly. Open the paper to reveal the mirror image of the face. The next stage is the lion's mane—again, it may be easier to draw this before painting. Fill in the triangles with paint, fold the paper in half, and open up to reveal the mane.

WHAT YOU WILL NEED

- ✪ plain paper
- ✪ pencil
- ✪ paint in your chosen colors
- ✪ paintbrushes in various sizes
- ✪ saucers to hold paint
- ✪ small pompom for lion's nose

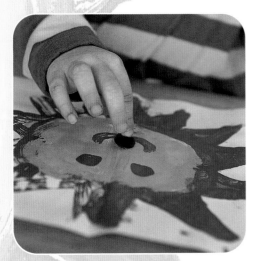

4 FINISHING Fill in one eye and half of the mouth using brown paint. Fold the paper in half, press it flat, and open to reveal the lion's face. As a finishing touch, we added a pompom for the lion's nose.

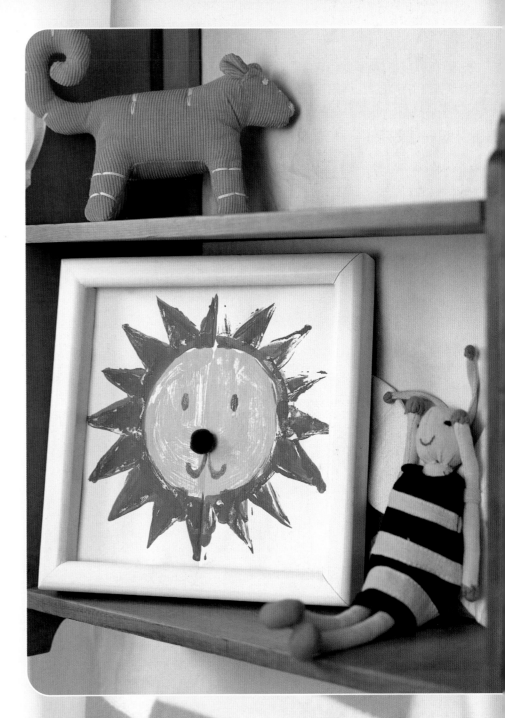

halloween hat

A simple cone of black card stock is the basis of this spooky witch's hat with a brim, or the simpler wizard's hat without a brim. Decorate with black net and silver stars for a night of trick-or-treating!

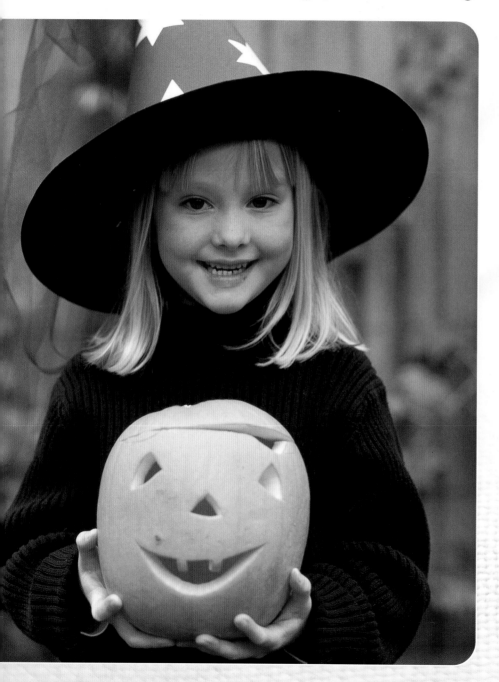

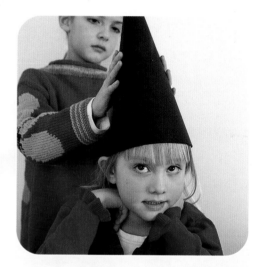

1 **MEASURE AND CUT** Cut out a semicircle of black card stock with a diameter of approximately 24in/60cm. Roll into a cone shape and fit to the child's head. Mark out the line where the card should be joined. Use strong tape to create the cone (we used black duct tape, which is the same color as the hat). A couple of staples will make the hat more secure.

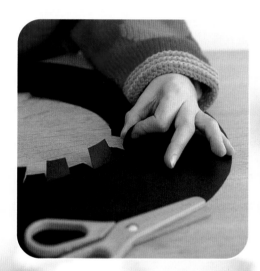

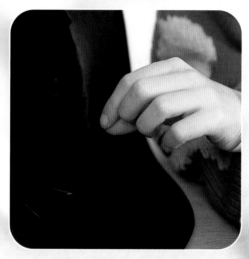

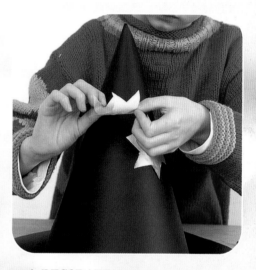

2 CUT OUT BRIM Place the cone on a sheet of black card stock and draw all the way around the opening. Then draw another larger circle about 3in/8cm wider, to form the brim. Mark a smaller circle 1in/2cm within the inner circle to allow for the flaps for the brim. Cut out the brim from the card. Use scissors to cut the flaps for the brim at intervals of 1in/ 2cm all the way around the inner circle.

3 ATTACH HAT AND BRIM Fold alternate flaps back and sit the cone on top of the brim. Use strong adhesive tape to fix the flaps to the cone. Firmly press down the tape to keep the brim in place.

4 DECORATE We used a star-shaped cookie cutter as a template to draw stars on silver paper. Cut them out with scissors and glue carefully to the hat. We also added a length of black netting, which we glued to the point of the hat as a finishing touch.

seed necklace

When it's too cold or wet to play outside, why not make your own jewelry from dried pumpkin seeds and sycamore wings threaded on cotton? It's a great way of using up the seeds from the Halloween jack o' lantern project on pages 104–105.

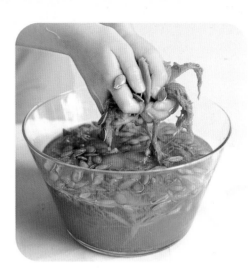

1 WASH SEEDS Using your hands or a spoon, scoop out the flesh and seeds from a pumpkin. Put all the seeds in a bowl of warm water and leave to soak for a couple of hours so that the flesh comes away from the seeds. Carefully pick out the seeds and place in a colander.

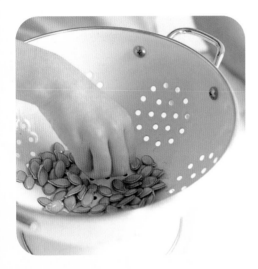

2 RINSE SEEDS When all the seeds are in the colander, run them under a tap to remove any bits of pumpkin flesh.

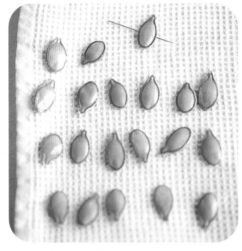

3 DRY AND PIERCE SEEDS Lay the seeds in rows on a tray covered with a clean dishcloth. Leave in a warm, dry place until the seeds have dried out. This can take up to a week. When the seeds are dry, use a needle to pierce holes through each seed ready for threading onto the necklace. It is advisable for an adult to carry out this task for younger children.

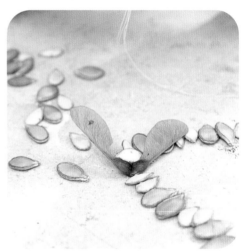

4 THREAD ON SEEDS Thread the cotton thread on the needle and knot the ends. Begin threading the seeds and intersperse them with sycamore wings. When threading is complete, tie the ends of the thread in a knot to finish.

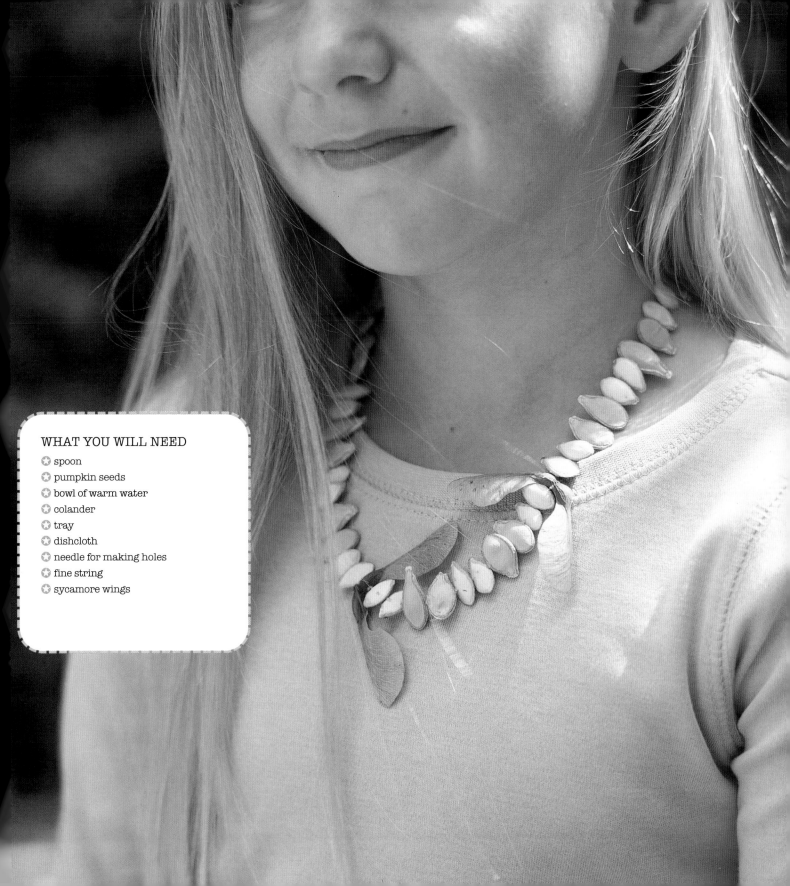

WHAT YOU WILL NEED

- ⭐ spoon
- ⭐ pumpkin seeds
- ⭐ bowl of warm water
- ⭐ colander
- ⭐ tray
- ⭐ dishcloth
- ⭐ needle for making holes
- ⭐ fine string
- ⭐ sycamore wings

pretty seed packets

It's fun and satisfying harvesting your own seeds and then packaging them up for the following year in these pretty decorated envelopes. You could also give them to family and friends.

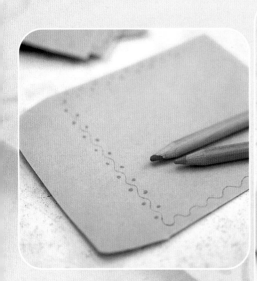

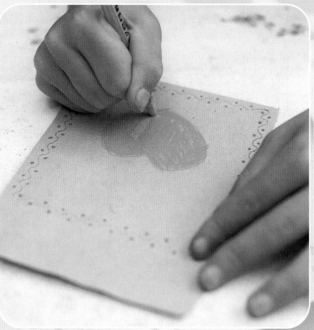

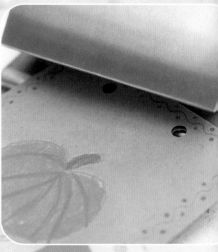

1 DECORATE ENVELOPE Using colored pencils, decorate the edges of the front of the envelope with pretty designs, such as wavy lines and and tiny polka dots.

2 DRAW ON DESIGN Using the colored pencils, draw the shape of a flower or vegetable, depending on what sort of seeds are in the envelope. You could add the name of the seeds in your best handwriting.

3 PUNCH HOLES Use a hole punch to make two holes at the top of the envelope, just where the flap is situated. Now carefully put the seeds in the envelope, and seal it closed.

WHAT YOU WILL NEED

- ✪ small brown envelopes
- ✪ colored pencils
- ✪ hole punch
- ✪ seeds
- ✪ 10in/25cm raffia ribbon per packet
- ✪ scissors

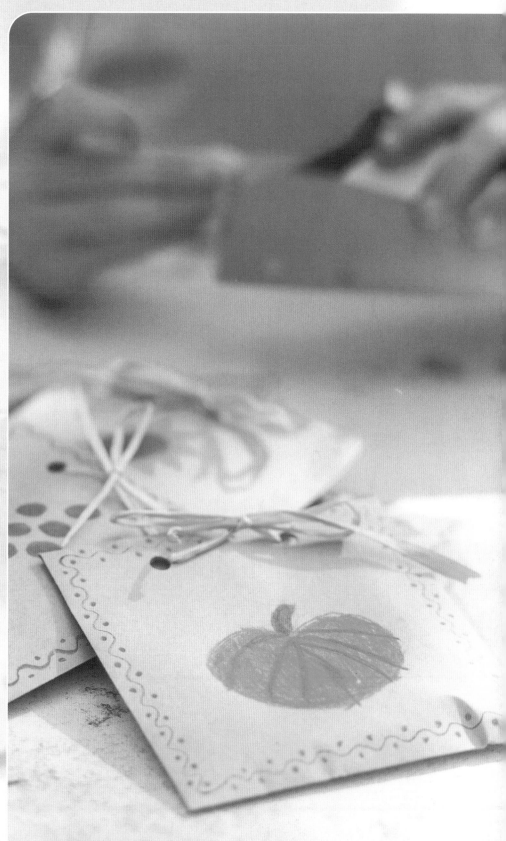

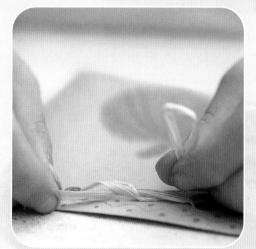

4 FINISHING Thread the raffia through the two punched holes and tie in a decorative bow. Trim the ends of the raffia with scissors to finish.

lavender bags

These simple but very pretty lavender bags are easy to sew and make lovely gifts for family and friends. We used a combination of a pastel-colored floral print and dotted cotton fabric to create vintage-style lavender bags.

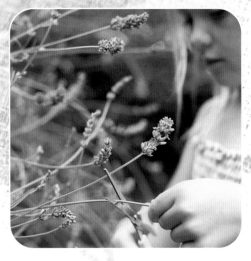

1 CUT AND DRY LAVENDER
Using scissors, carefully snip off long stems of lavender. Cover a tray with a sheet of waxed paper and place the lavender on top to dry. Put the tray in a warm, dry place until the herbs have dried completely. Carefully pull off the lavender heads by hand and collect them in a bowl .

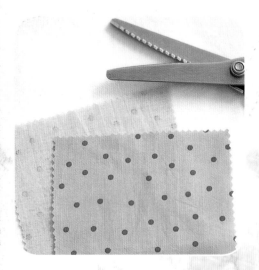

2 CUT OUT THE BAGS
Using pinking shears to prevent the fabric from fraying, cut a rectangle of fabric measuring 5 x 8in/12 x 20cm, or two rectangles of 5 x 16in/12 x 40cm.

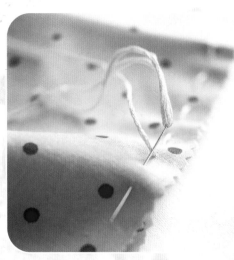

3 STITCH BAGS
With wrong sides facing, stitch together the sides of the fabric (and the base of the bag, if you are using two pieces of fabric) using running stitch and contrasting colored cotton embroidery thread. The stitches should be no more than ½in/1cm apart, so the lavender cannot leak out.

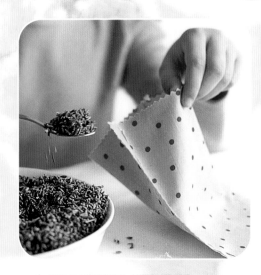

4 FILL WITH LAVENDER
When the bag is complete, use a teaspoon to carefully fill it with loose lavender. Fill the bag to approximately halfway up, and make sure it is quite plump and full.

5 FINISHING Lay the lavender bag on one side and wrap the cotton ribbon around the bag, just above the lavender. Tie a bow, then trim the ends using scissors.

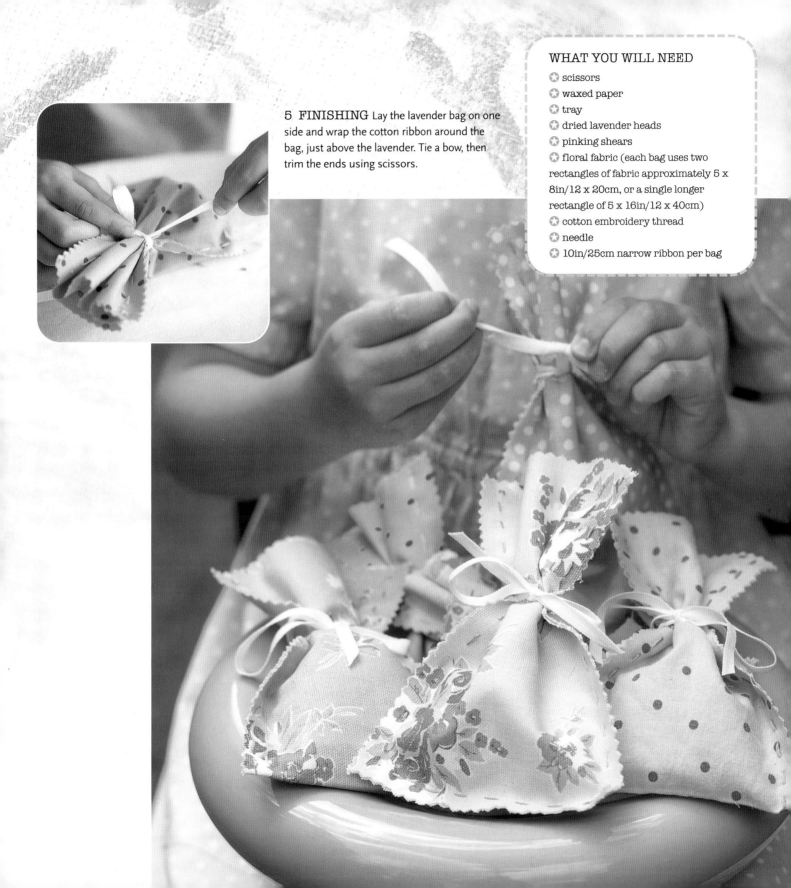

jack o' lantern

This carved Halloween pumpkin looks more friendly than spooky! He's been given a pointy parsnip nose and a thick head of carrot-frond "hair." Fill him with tealights and leave him by the door to greet trick-or-treaters.

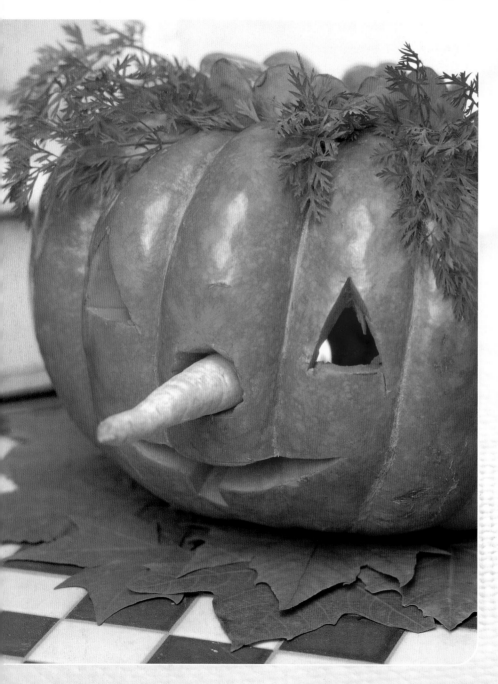

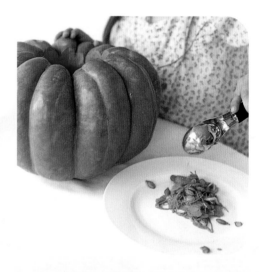

1 SCOOP OUT SEEDS Ask an adult to cut the top off the pumpkin using a sharp knife. Scoop out the flesh and seeds using an ice-cream scoop or a large spoon.

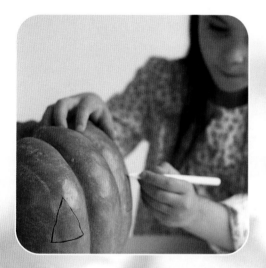

2 DRAW ON FACE Draw eyes, nose and a mouth onto the pumpkin using a marker pen. Ask an adult to cut out the shapes using a sharp knife.

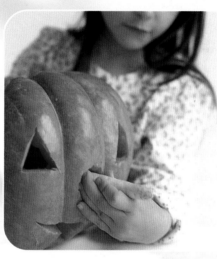

3 INSERT NOSE Push the thick end of the parsnip into the nose hole to make a pointy nose. Cut the fronds from the carrots to prepare the hair.

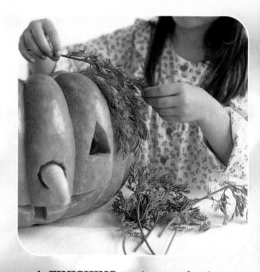

4 FINISHING Lay the carrot fronds around the top of the pumpkin to make the hair. Place two or three tealights inside the pumpkin and ask an adult to light them. Now place the pumpkin by the front door.

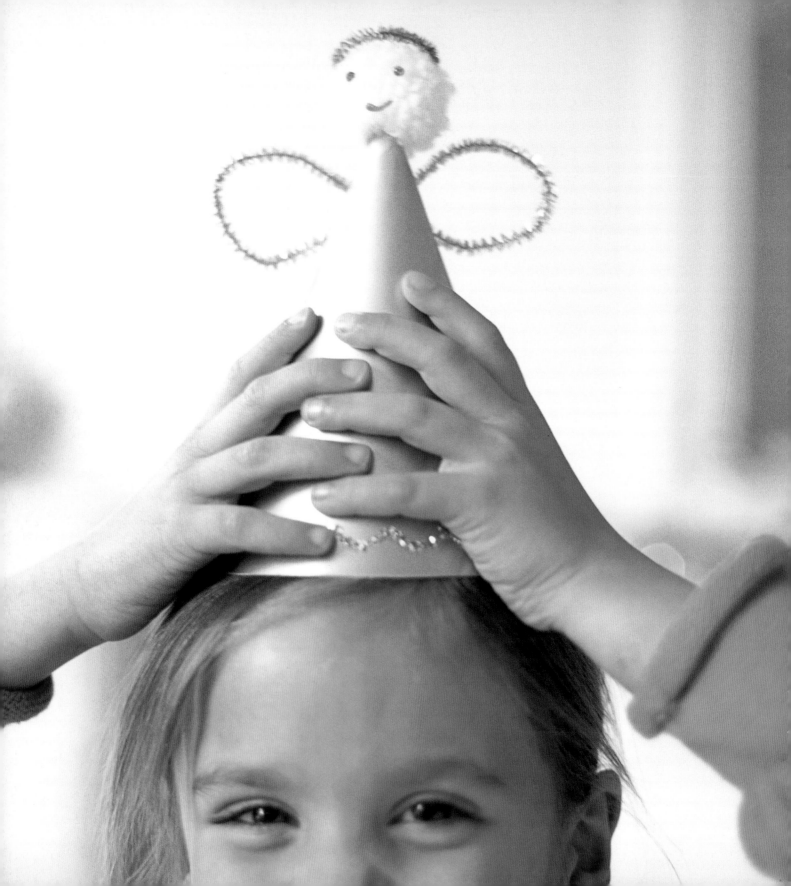

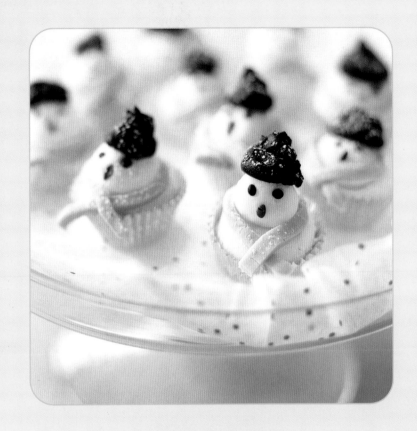

winter

twig decorations

These delicate-looking star decorations are crafted from thin twigs gathered from the garden or the park, painted silver and then tied together with fine wire. The twig stars look so pretty dangling in a row from a mantelpiece or hung in clusters on a Christmas tree.

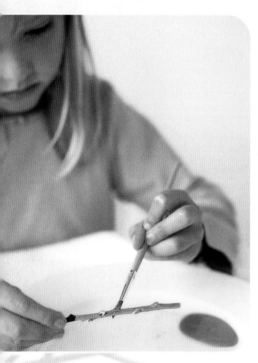

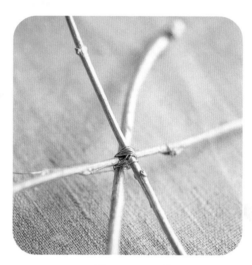

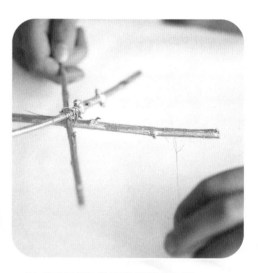

1 APPLY PAINT Choose three 4in-/10cm-long twigs and paint them silver. Allow to dry thoroughly. If required, apply a second coat of paint for better coverage and leave to dry.

2 FORM STAR SHAPE Lay the three twigs one on top of each other to form a star shape. Cut a length of fine wire and bind it round the twigs to hold the star in place. Wrap the wire over the twigs several times, so that they are completely secure.

3 ATTACH HANGING LOOP Cut a length of thread for the hanging loop and fold it in half. Wrap it round one "arm" of the star, thread the ends back through the loop, and pull to attach the thread to the twig. Knot the two loose ends together to form a hanging loop.

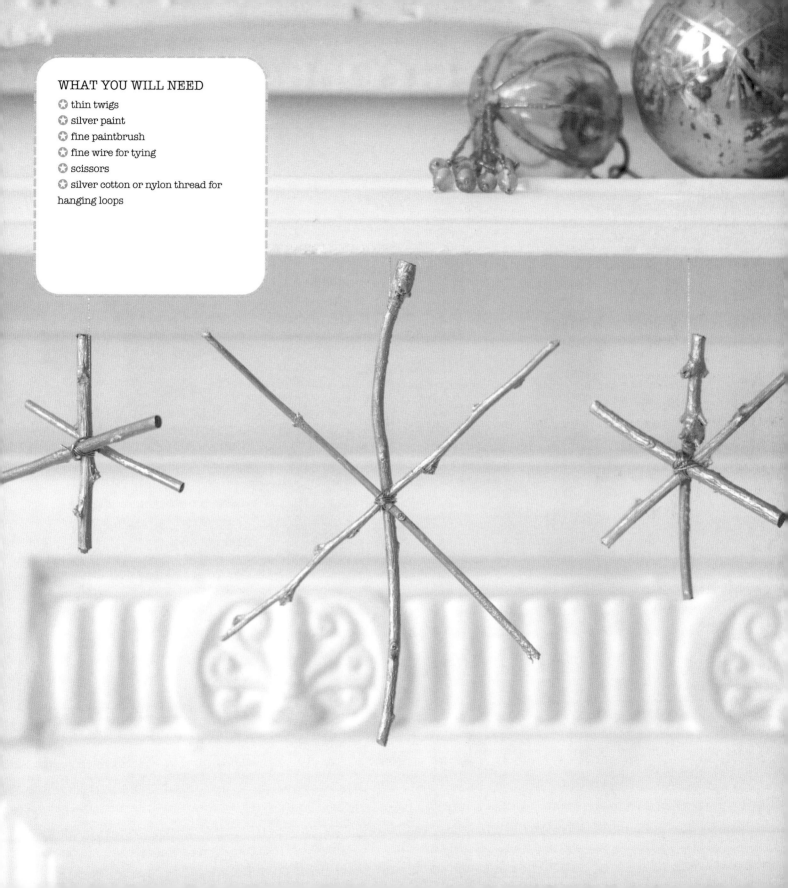

WHAT YOU WILL NEED

✪ thin twigs

✪ silver paint

✪ fine paintbrush

✪ fine wire for tying

✪ scissors

✪ silver cotton or nylon thread for hanging loops

orange tree decorations

Dried orange slices hung from a pretty gingham ribbon loop make fragrant and unusual Christmas tree decorations. They also make a great addition to our potpourri, which can be found on pages 124-125.

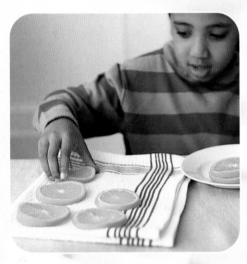

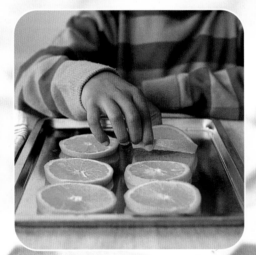

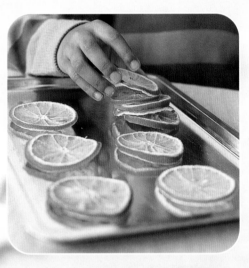

1 SLICE THE ORANGES Ask an adult to cut the orange into slices that are approximately ¼in/5mm wide. Now put the slices on a dishcloth and gently blot them with paper towels to remove any excess moisture. This should speed up the drying process.

2 BAKE IN OVEN Lay the orange slices on a metal baking sheet. Put them in the oven on the very lowest setting and leave them for about four hours or until they are completely dry. The trick is to let them "cook" long enough to dry completely. If the orange slices do not dry entirely, they won't keep for long and may even go moldy. Ask an adult to remove the sheet from the oven, as it will be very hot.

3 REMOVE DRIED ORANGES Once the tray has completely cooled, remove the orange slices from the tray and set them aside for decorating. The slices should be hard and dry, but retain their delicious citrus fragrance.

WHAT YOU WILL NEED

- ✿ fresh oranges
- ✿ sharp knife
- ✿ dishcloth
- ✿ paper towels
- ✿ baking sheet
- ✿ wooden skewer or awl
- ✿ 6in/15cm gingham ribbon (½in/1cm wide) for each hanging loop

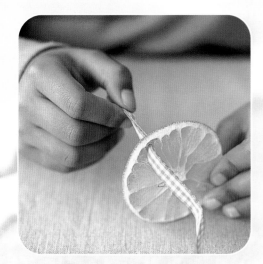

4 FINISHING Ask an adult to make a small hole in the orange using a sharp point such as a wooden skewer. Thread the ribbon through the hole and tie the ends in a knot. Trim the ribbon ends on the diagonal to prevent them from fraying.

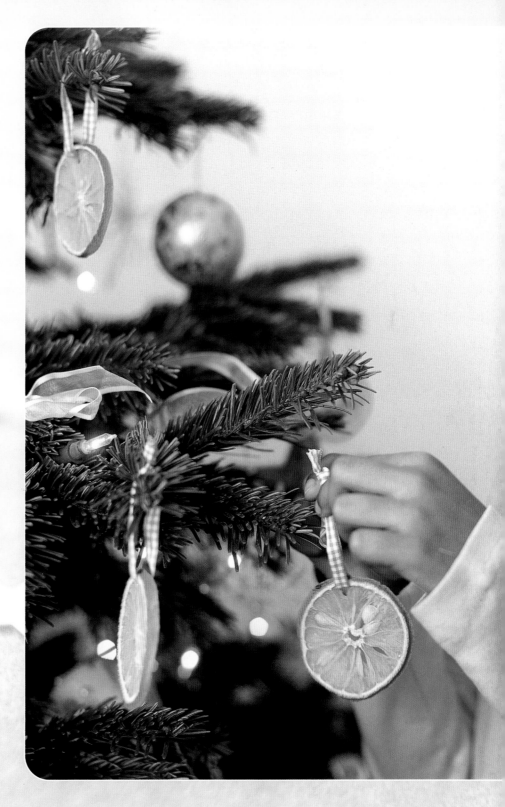

paper snowflakes

Paper snowflakes are so simple to make, yet so effective. Cut them from white paper, tissue paper, or tracing paper to create pretty and inexpensive Christmas decorations. They can be used to decorate windows or suspended from lengths of cotton for a mobile effect.

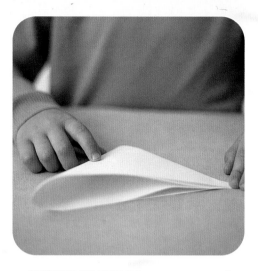

1 FOLD PAPER Take a square piece of paper. Fold it in half diagonally to form a triangle. Then fold in half again and then into quarters. You should now have a small folded triangle shape.

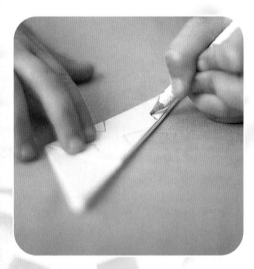

2 DRAW ON DESIGN Using the pencil, draw triangular or scalloped designs on the folded edges of the paper. You can draw curved shapes on the top edges of the paper (furthest from the center), too. Experiment with different shapes, so that all your snowflakes are slightly different.

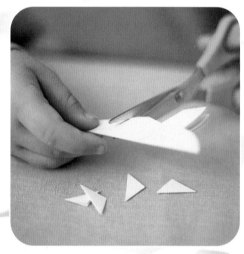

3 CUT OUT Using scissors, carefully cut along the lines you have drawn on the paper. The more shapes you cut out, the more decorative and delicate your finished snowflake will be.

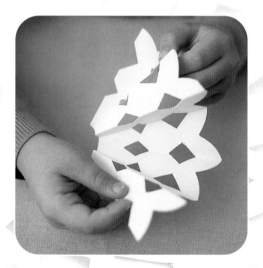

4 PULL OPEN Gently unfold the paper and carefully press it flat to reveal the snowflake's design. You can cut snowflakes from any piece of paper, but good sizes are an 8in/20cm square for a large snowflake and a 4in/10cm square for a small one.

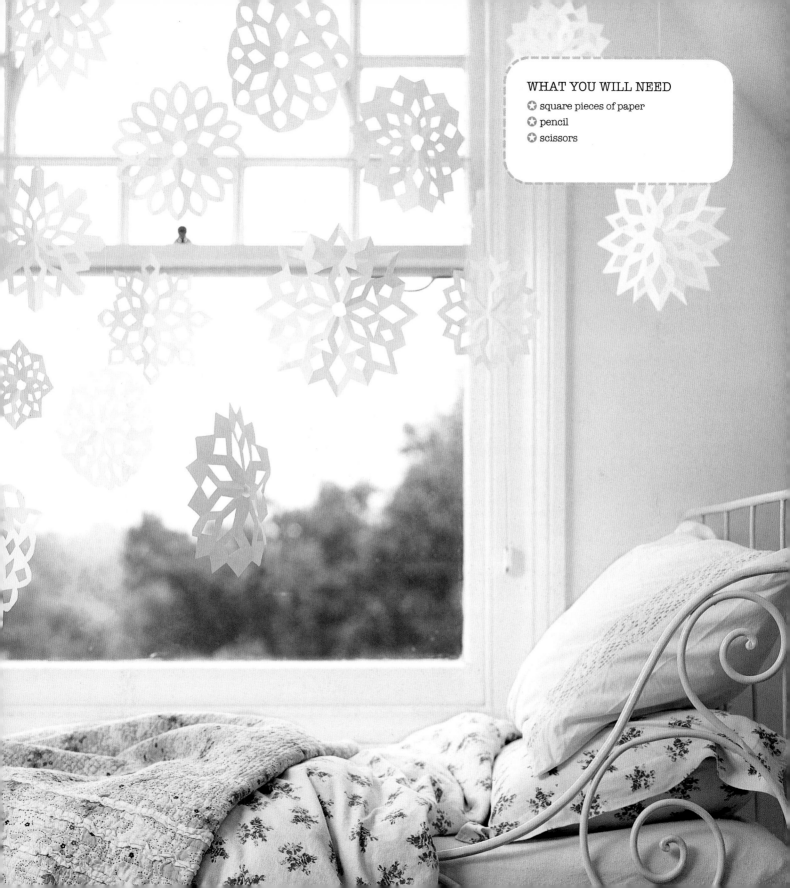

pine cone animals

These cute animals are crafted from pine cones and are decorated with felt ears, pompom eyes, and curly pipe-cleaner tails. Different-sized pine cones will lend themselves to different creatures!

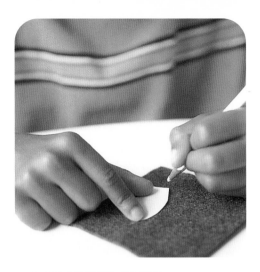

1 DRAW EAR SHAPE Draw an ear shape onto paper and cut out with scissors to make a template. Place the template on the felt and draw around it. Repeat for the second ear.

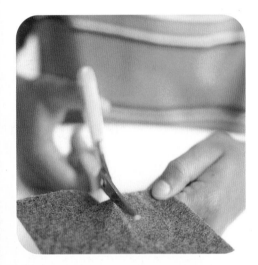

2 CUT AND GLUE EARS Carefully cut out the ears. Pinch each one in half and put a dab of glue inside the fold to form a pleat. Allow to dry.

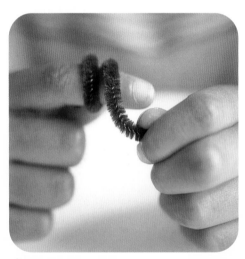

3 MAKE TAIL Cut a piece of pipe-cleaner approximately 4in/10cm long and wind it around a finger to create a tail.

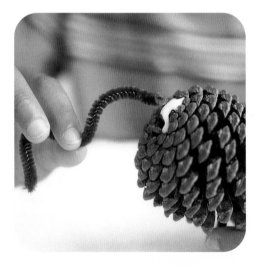

4 GLUE ON TAIL Apply a dab of glue to the base of the pine cone and stick the tail to this. Press down gently to ensure that the tail is securely in position, and leave to dry completely.

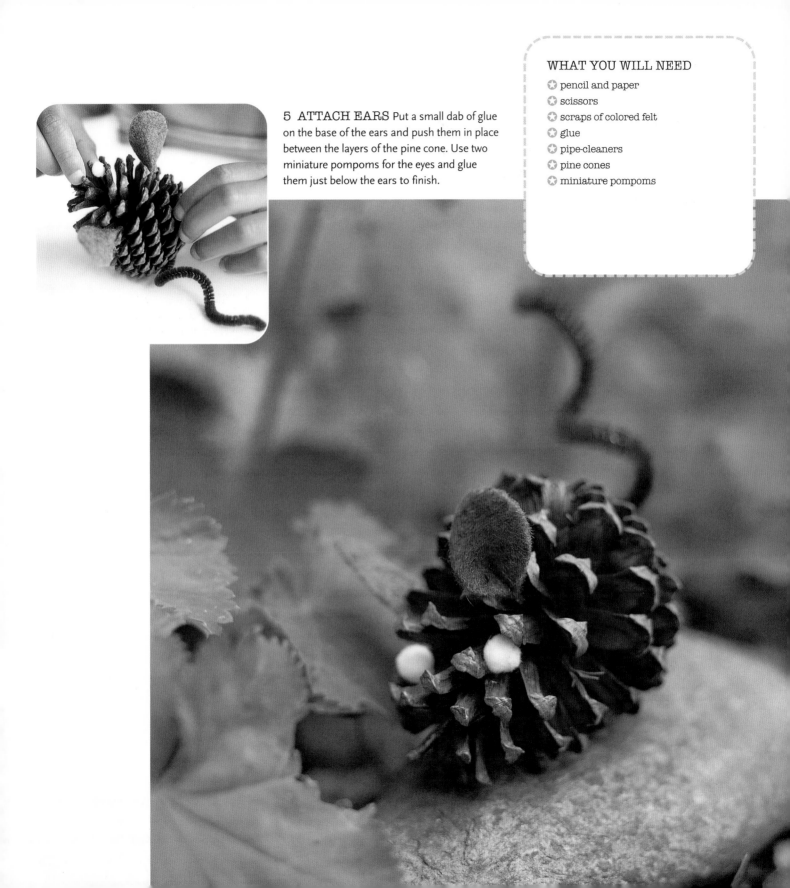

5 ATTACH EARS Put a small dab of glue on the base of the ears and push them in place between the layers of the pine cone. Use two miniature pompoms for the eyes and glue them just below the ears to finish.

WHAT YOU WILL NEED

- ✪ pencil and paper
- ✪ scissors
- ✪ scraps of colored felt
- ✪ glue
- ✪ pipe-cleaners
- ✪ pine cones
- ✪ miniature pompoms

paper chains

Traditional paper chains are so easy to make, and look fantastic at children's parties or other celebrations. We used a combination of zingy hot pinks and oranges, but you could try making paper chains in soft pastel tones or in red and white to use as Christmas decorations.

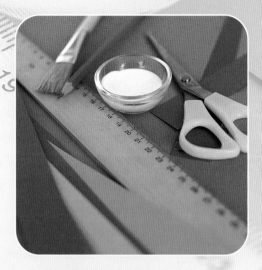

1 CHOOSE COLORS Ask your child what colors she or he would like to use to create the chains. For more decorative paper chains, you could use patterned gift wrap or translucent tracing paper, which is available from art shops in a variety of different colors.

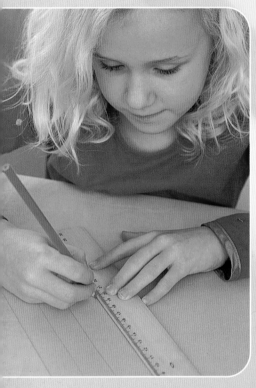

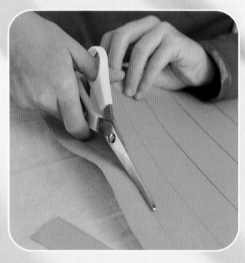

2 DRAW STRIPS Using a pencil and ruler, draw the strips on the back of the paper, making sure that each one is approximately 1in/2cm wide.

3 CUT STRIPS Using scissors, cut out the strips. It is a good idea to keep the colors separate by making a pile of strips in each color, so they are easier to select when joining the chains together.

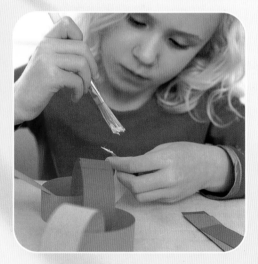

4 GLUE STRIPS INTO CHAINS Form a loop with the first paper chain and put a dab of glue on one end to stick it together. For the next link, thread the paper through the loop and glue the ends. Repeat to make more links, until you have made the required length of paper chain.

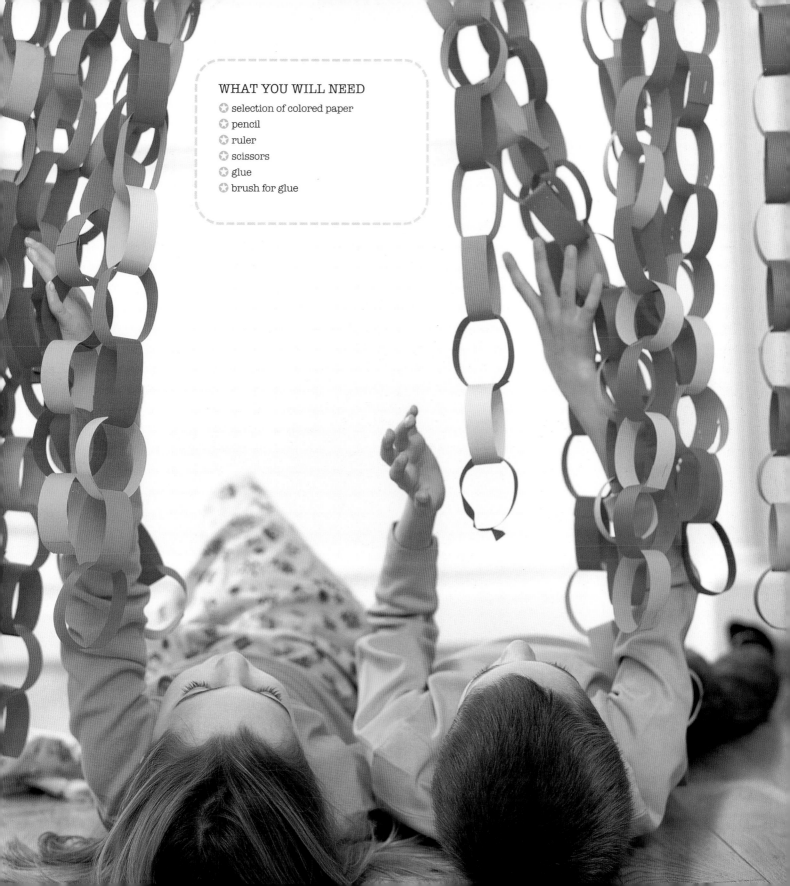

WHAT YOU WILL NEED

- ✪ selection of colored paper
- ✪ pencil
- ✪ ruler
- ✪ scissors
- ✪ glue
- ✪ brush for glue

finger- and hand-painting

Any painting undertaken in our house inevitably ends up with the children painting parts of themselves too, so a project that requires them to paint themselves is guaranteed to be popular. Paint-and-bake ceramic kits that can be "fired" in a domestic oven can be bought from many craft suppliers, and are ideal for this project.

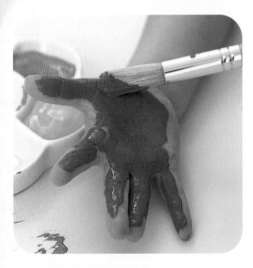

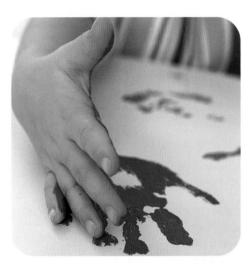

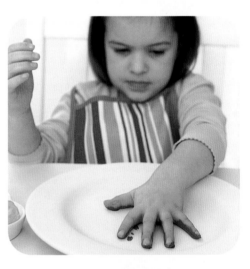

1 PAINT HANDS In separate saucers or on a paint tray, put out a small amount of each of the paints to be used. Use a thick brush to apply the paint to the palm of the hand. Make sure the paint is not too thick. Keep a cloth to hand in case of accidents.

2 PRACTICE PRINTING Before attempting to decorate your plate, help your child practice their technique. The hand needs to be pressed as flat as possible, with the fingers slightly splayed to show the shape. Once the printing technique has been mastered on paper, you can move on to the real thing.

3 PRINT ON PLATE Clean off any excess paint from the practice run, and reapply fresh paint to the hand. Use one color, or paint different fingers in different colors. Press the hand flat with fingers splayed, as before. Carefully lift the hand off the plate and allow the paint to dry.

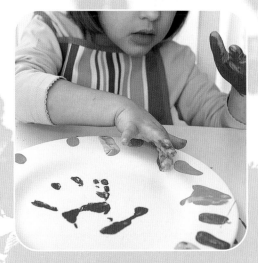

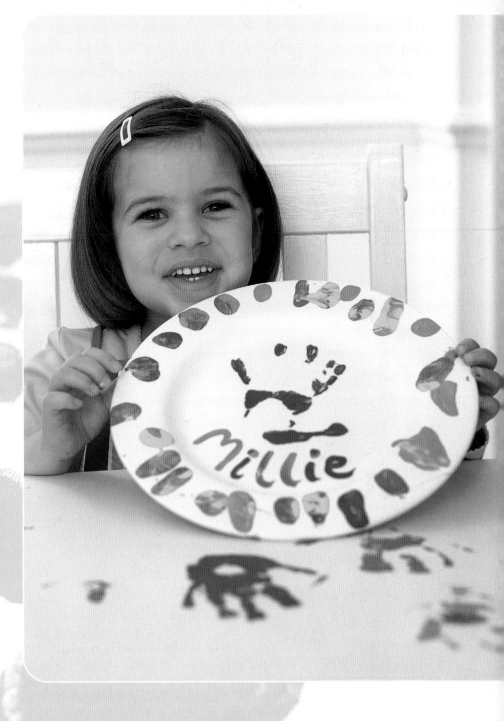

4 FINISHING Apply a coat of paint to the fingertips and print around the edge of the plate to create a border. The child may also like to write his or her name on the plate. To fix the paint, bake the item in the oven, following the manufacturer's instructions, or take it to a pottery café to have it fired in the kiln.

felt motif cards

Felt is great for decorating cards as it comes in a wide selection of colors and does not fray once it is cut. We used Christmas-themed cookie cutters as templates for a variety of festive designs. Glue the felt shapes onto cardboard and finish them with dainty ribbon bows.

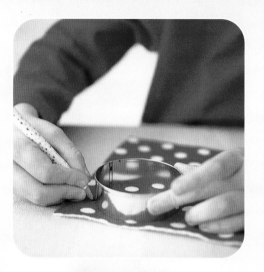

1 CUT OUT FELT MOTIF Use the circular cookie cutter (or a similar object) as a template for the round shape on this card. Place it on the felt and draw around it with a pencil. Carefully cut out the round shape. If you are making more than one card, it's a good idea to cut out all your felt shapes at the same time.

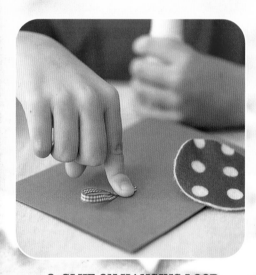

2 GLUE ON HANGING LOOP Cut a piece of gingham ribbon about 2in/5cm long and fold it into a loop. Glue the ribbon onto the card. Press down firmly to fix it in place.

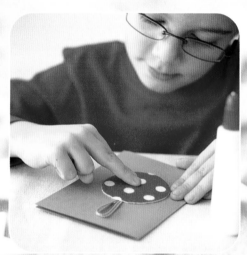

3 STICK ON FELT SHAPE Apply a thin layer of glue to the back of the felt shape and stick it onto the card, making sure that you have concealed the ends of the ribbon loop. Press down firmly and allow to dry completely.

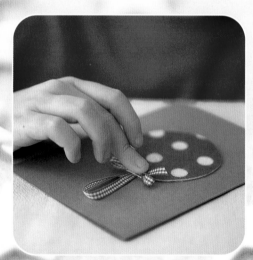

4 FINISHING Make a ribbon bow from the gingham ribbon. Apply a tiny dab of glue to the back of the bow, and stick to the front of the felt motif. Press down firmly to secure it in place and leave to dry.

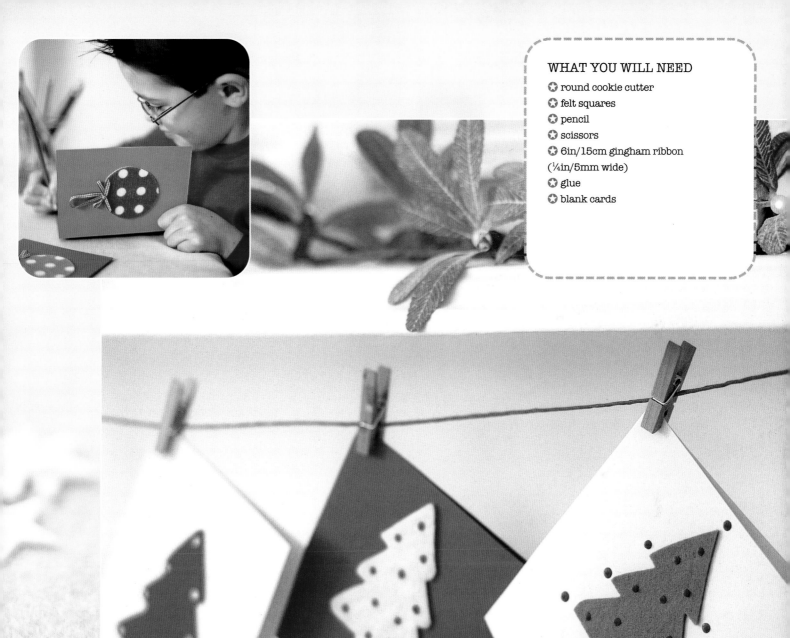

WHAT YOU WILL NEED

⭐ round cookie cutter
⭐ felt squares
⭐ pencil
⭐ scissors
⭐ 6in/15cm gingham ribbon
(¼in/5mm wide)
⭐ glue
⭐ blank cards

peppermint creams

Delicious to eat and oh-so-easy to make, peppermint creams make great gifts and the mixture can be used to form fun shapes, such as these cute snowmen with their black icing hats and snug blue scarves!

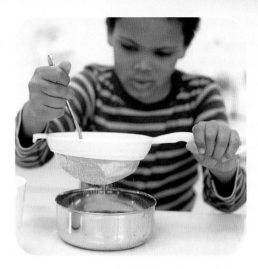

1 MIX INGREDIENTS Sift the sugar into a bowl and stir in the condensed milk until the mixture becomes a smooth paste. Add three drops of oil of peppermint and knead it into the mixture until the flavour is thoroughly worked through. Add more oil of peppermint a drop at a time and knead it in thoroughly until you achieve the desired intensity of flavour.

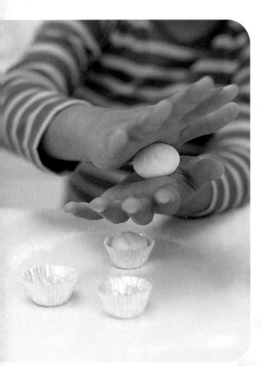

2 FORM SNOWMEN Roll the mixture between the palms of your hands to form a ball for the bottom half of the snowman. Place in a petit-four case, then roll a smaller ball for the head. Place the head gently on top of the larger ball and push down gently so the balls stick to each other.

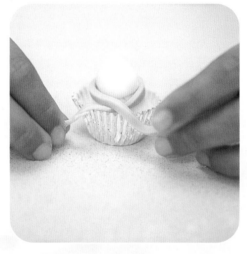

3 ADD SCARVES Roll out the pale blue icing. Ask an adult to use a sharp knife to cut lengths measuring about 1/4in/5mm wide by 4in/10cm long. Wrap one around the neck of each snowman to form a scarf.

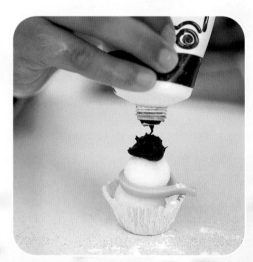

4 FINISHING Use ready-mixed black icing to form the snowmen's hats and eyes. To finish, roll blobs of brown icing into tiny balls for the snowmen's noses and stick them firmly in place. Let the snowmen dry completely before packaging them up.

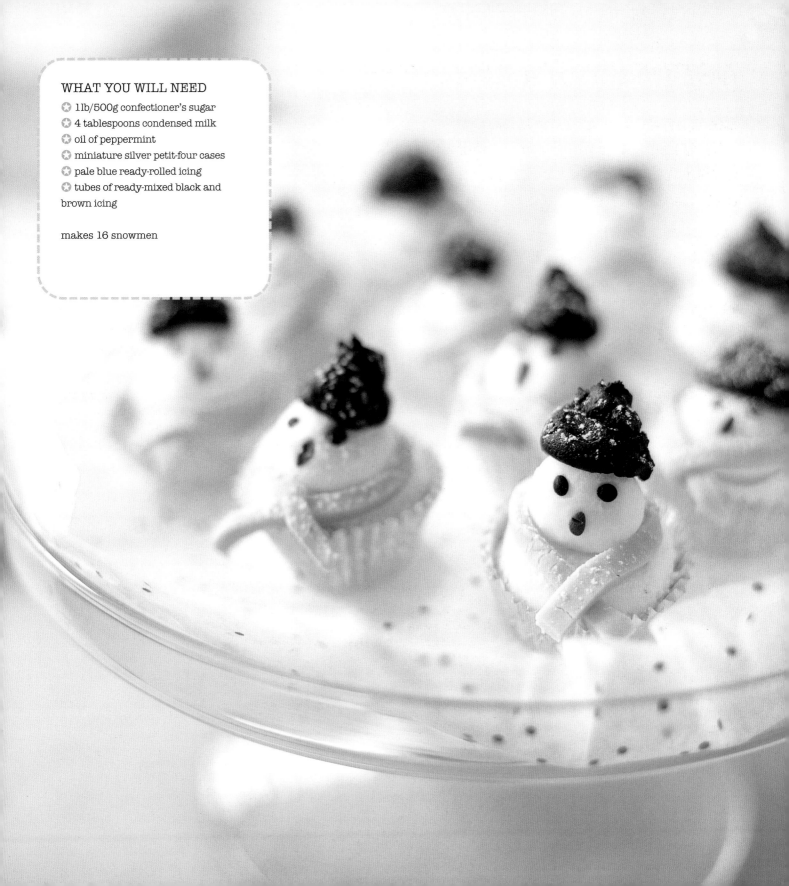

WHAT YOU WILL NEED

- 1lb/500g confectioner's sugar
- 4 tablespoons condensed milk
- oil of peppermint
- miniature silver petit-four cases
- pale blue ready-rolled icing
- tubes of ready-mixed black and brown icing

makes 16 snowmen

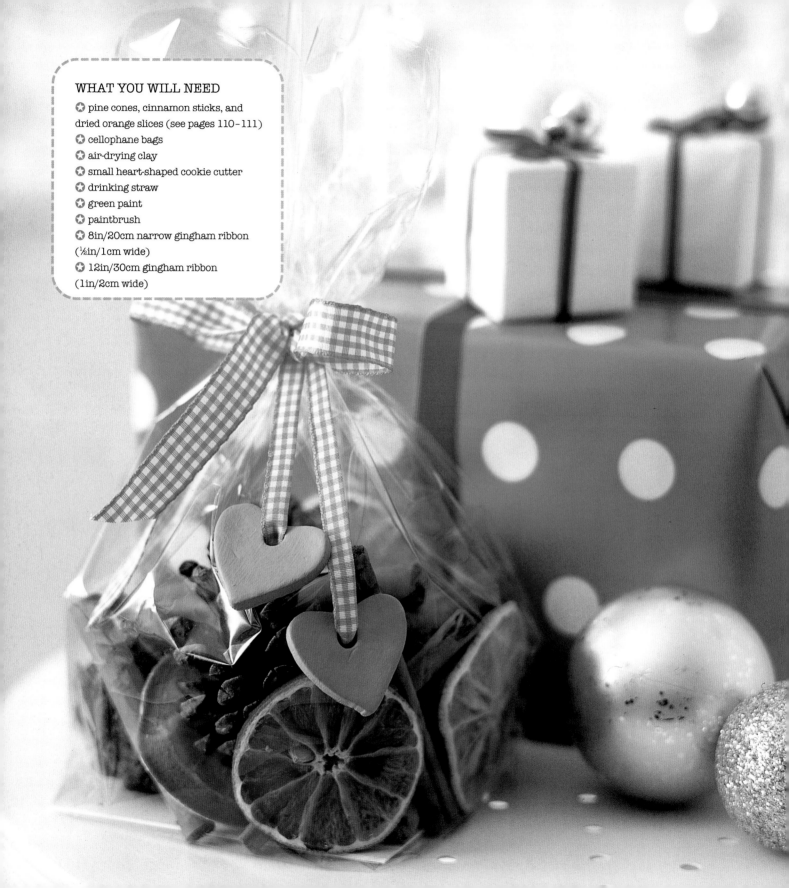

WHAT YOU WILL NEED

✪ pine cones, cinnamon sticks, and
dried orange slices (see pages 110–111)

✪ cellophane bags

✪ air-drying clay

✪ small heart-shaped cookie cutter

✪ drinking straw

✪ green paint

✪ paintbrush

✪ 8in/20cm narrow gingham ribbon
(½in/1cm wide)

✪ 12in/30cm gingham ribbon
(1in/2cm wide)

potpourri

Sweetly scented potpourri is fun and easy to make and is always a welcome gift. It looks very pretty packaged in a glossy cellophane bag and decorated with ribbon and little heart-shaped clay decorations.

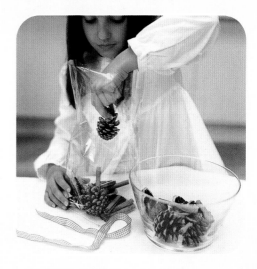

1 FILL BAG Make the dried orange slices following the instructions on pages 110–111. Put the cones, cinnamon sticks, and orange slices into a bowl. Now fill the cellophane bag with the potpourri, layering the different items for an attractive effect.

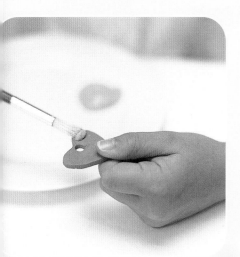

2 PAINT CLAY DECORATIONS Following the instructions on pages 86–87, make two clay hearts per bag of potpourri. Use a heart-shaped cookie cutter to cut them out, and use a drinking straw to pierce a hole in each one to thread the ribbon through. Let dry, then paint the hearts green on both sides.

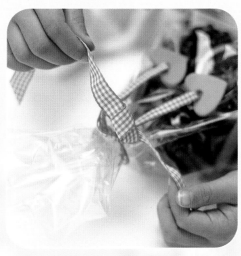

3 TIE ON CLAY DECORATIONS Thread the narrow ribbon through the holes of one heart and tie a knot at the back of the heart to prevent it slipping off. Tie the narrow ribbon around the neck of the bag and draw tight. Now tie the thicker ribbon together around the ends of the narrow ribbon, just below the knot.

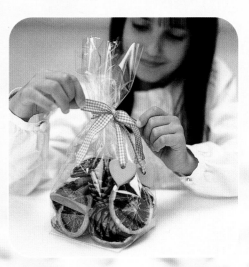

4 FINISHING Tie the thicker ribbon in a bow around the neck of the bag. Tease up the top of the bag so that it looks attractive. Trim the ends of the ribbon on the diagonal to prevent the ends from fraying.

holiday spice cookies

It's lots of fun making your own edible holiday decorations or treats for a special birthday party. Just cut shapes out of a sweet cookie dough, then have lots of fun decorating them with colored icing and silver balls.

WHAT YOU WILL NEED
⭐ 2 non-stick cookie sheets
⭐ 1½ sticks/175g unsalted butter, straight from the fridge, plus extra butter for greasing
⭐ 2⅓ cups/300g all-purpose flour
⭐ 2 teaspoons ground cinnamon
⭐ ½ teaspoon ground ginger
⭐ ½ teaspoon ground apple-pie spice
⭐ 6 tablespoons clear honey
⭐ thin ribbon, thread, or raffia, to hang
⭐ icing pens and silver balls, to decorate
⭐ a selection of shaped cookie cutters such as stars, Christmas trees, angels, bells, and reindeer

makes about 24 cookies

1 Put a bit of butter on a piece of paper towel and rub it on the baking sheets to grease them.

2 Put the flour, cinnamon, ginger, and apple-pie spice in the bowl of a food processor. Using an ordinary table knife, cut the butter into small pieces and add to the bowl of the processor.

3 Ask an adult to help you run the processor until the mixture looks like fine crumbs.

4 Measure the honey into the bowl of the processor and, with adult help, run the processor until the mixture comes together to make a ball of dough.

5 Ask an adult to help you remove the blade from the bowl, then remove the dough from the bowl. Wrap the dough in plastic wrap or waxed paper and put it into the fridge until it is firm enough to roll out—probably about 30 minutes.

6 Ask an adult to help you preheat the oven to 350°F/180°C.

7 Lightly sprinkle the work surface and a rolling pin with flour. Gently roll out the dough until it is about ¼in/5mm thick. Cut out shapes using your cookie cutters. Gather up the trimmings into a ball, then roll out and cut more shapes. To make Christmas decorations to hang up, you'll need to make a small hole at the top of each cookie with a wooden skewer (make sure it's large enough to thread a ribbon through).

8 Arrange the shapes slightly apart on the prepared baking sheets. Ask an adult to help you put them in the oven to bake for about 10 minutes, or until golden. Ask an adult to help you carefully remove them from the oven, put the trays onto a heatproof surface, and leave to cool for 5 minutes. Gently transfer the cookies to a wire rack and leave until cold.

9 Decorate the cookies however you like; you could thread them with ribbon, then ice using icing pens and silver balls. Leave until the icing is set, then hang them up. Eat your cookies as soon as possible, or store them in an airtight container and eat within five days.

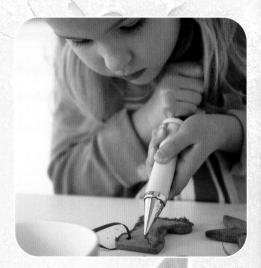

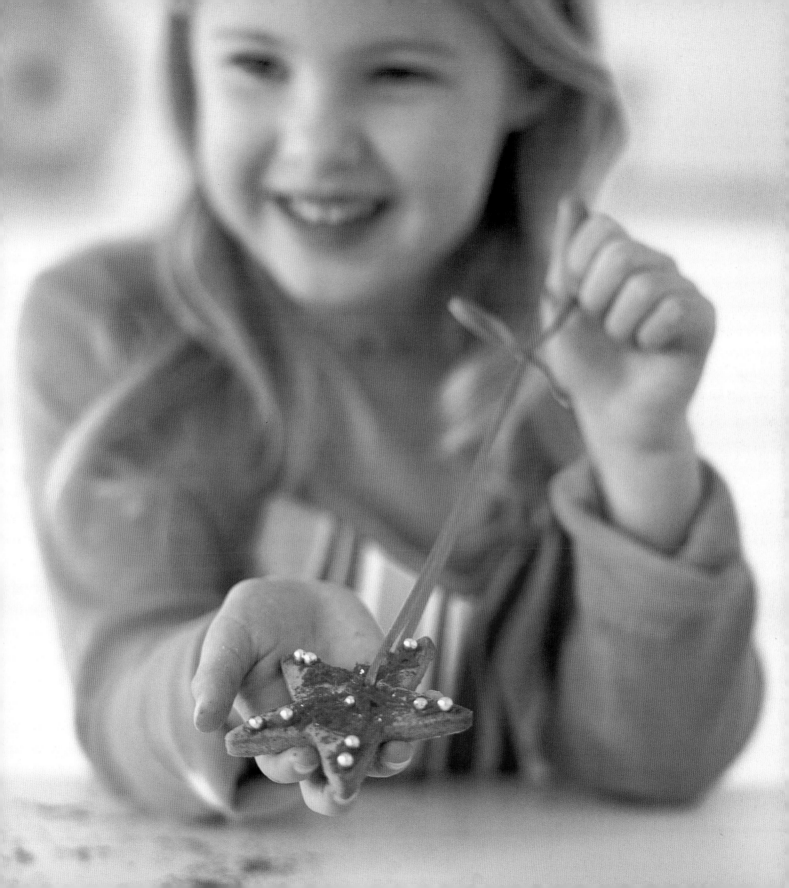

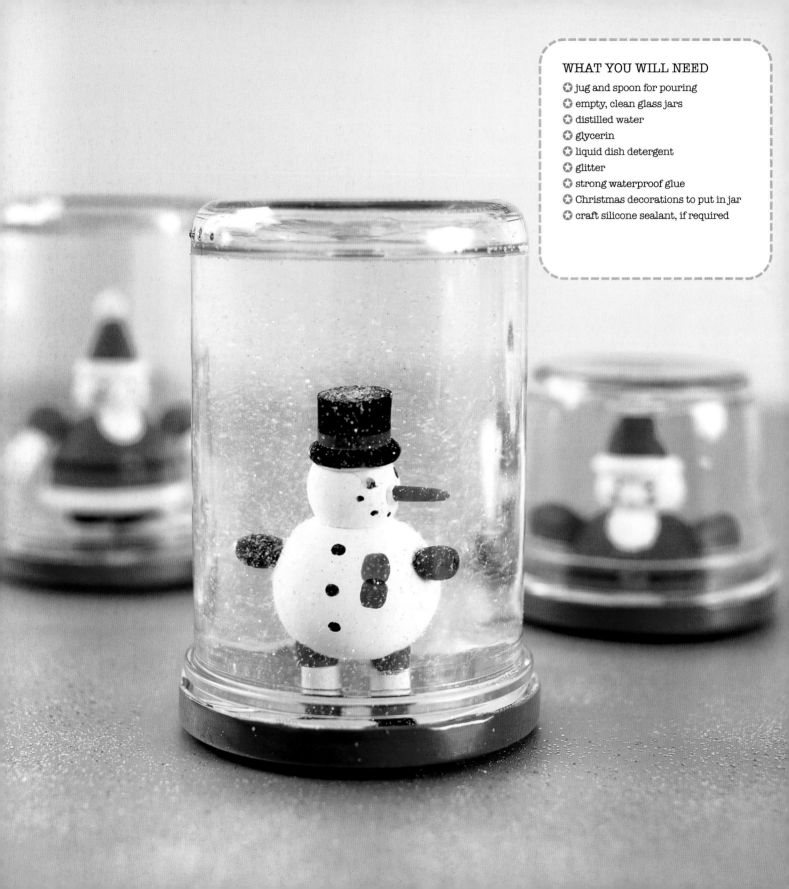

WHAT YOU WILL NEED

- ✪ jug and spoon for pouring
- ✪ empty, clean glass jars
- ✪ distilled water
- ✪ glycerin
- ✪ liquid dish detergent
- ✪ glitter
- ✪ strong waterproof glue
- ✪ Christmas decorations to put in jar
- ✪ craft silicone sealant, if required

snow globes

Snow globes make great gifts and children always enjoy making them. We used Christmas decorations inside ours, but your child may like to use small plastic animals or even to make their own decorations to put inside.

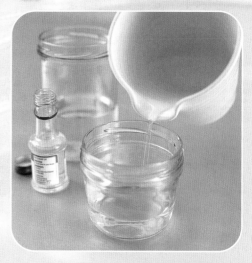

1 FILL JAR Use a jug to pour the distilled water into the glass jar. Fill it as full as possible. Add two teaspoons of glycerin and half a teaspoon of detergent.

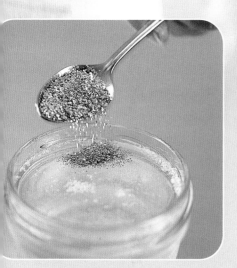

2 ADD GLITTER Spoon the glitter into the water. You will need approximately five or six teaspoons. White or silver glitter looks most similar to snow, although red or green or other bright colors look very festive.

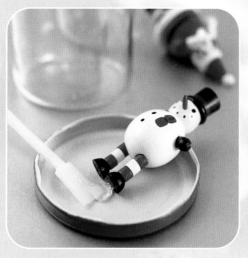

3 ATTACH DECORATION Use a blob of strong waterproof glue to securely attach the decoration to the inside of the jar lid. It is advisable for an adult to do this. Allow the glue to dry thoroughly according to the manufacturer's instructions.

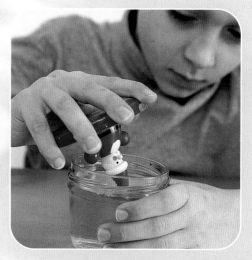

4 SECURE LID Carefully place the lid on the top of the jar and screw tightly in place. The jar should be watertight, but you may wish to seal it around the edges with a layer of craft silicone sealant, which is available from craft stores.

potato print wrapping paper

Potato printing is a traditional painting technique that is a favorite with kids of all ages. They can use cookie cutters to create pretty shapes, or an adult could use a sharp knife to cut out different shapes by hand.

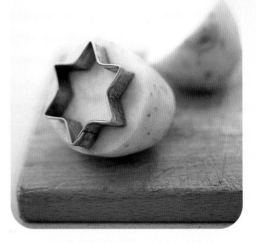

1 CUT OUT SHAPE Cut the potato in half, making sure the surface of the potato is as flat as possible. Place the cookie cutter on a cutting board with the sharp edge facing upward. Press the potato firmly down onto the cutter, leaving the cookie cutter standing proud of the cut surface of the potato by about ¼in/5mm, so you can cut all the way around it.

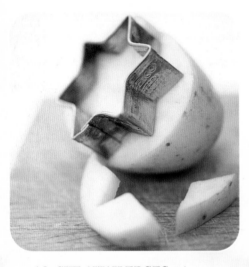

2 CUT AWAY EDGES Ask an adult to cut away the edges of the potato using a sharp knife. This needs to be done very carefully, to make sure the star shape is as clear as possible. Press the potato down on a paper towel or a dry cloth to remove any excess moisture, which can make the paint watery.

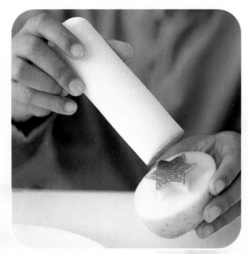

3 APPLY PAINT Pour paint into a saucer and use the end of the sponge roller to apply the paint to the star shape. Don't apply too much paint to the potato, as this will make the design bleed. If you have applied too much, gently blot the potato on a paper towel to remove the excess.

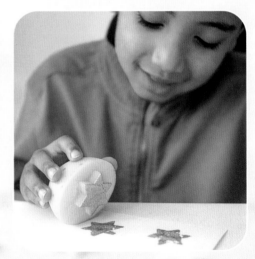

4 GET PRINTING Begin printing. To make sure the design prints clearly, use a gentle rocking motion, moving the potato from side to side without lifting it from the paper. This will apply the paint evenly, even if the cut surface of the potato is not flat. Continue to print the stars at evenly spaced intervals. Allow the paint to dry completely.

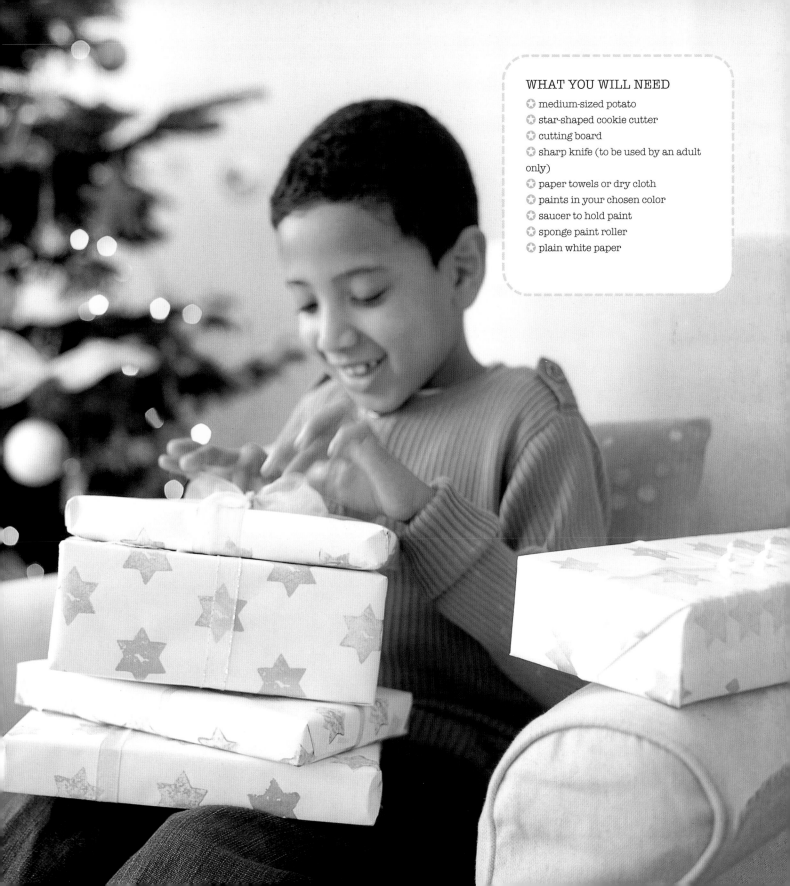

WHAT YOU WILL NEED

- ✪ medium-sized potato
- ✪ star-shaped cookie cutter
- ✪ cutting board
- ✪ sharp knife (to be used by an adult only)
- ✪ paper towels or dry cloth
- ✪ paints in your chosen color
- ✪ saucer to hold paint
- ✪ sponge paint roller
- ✪ plain white paper

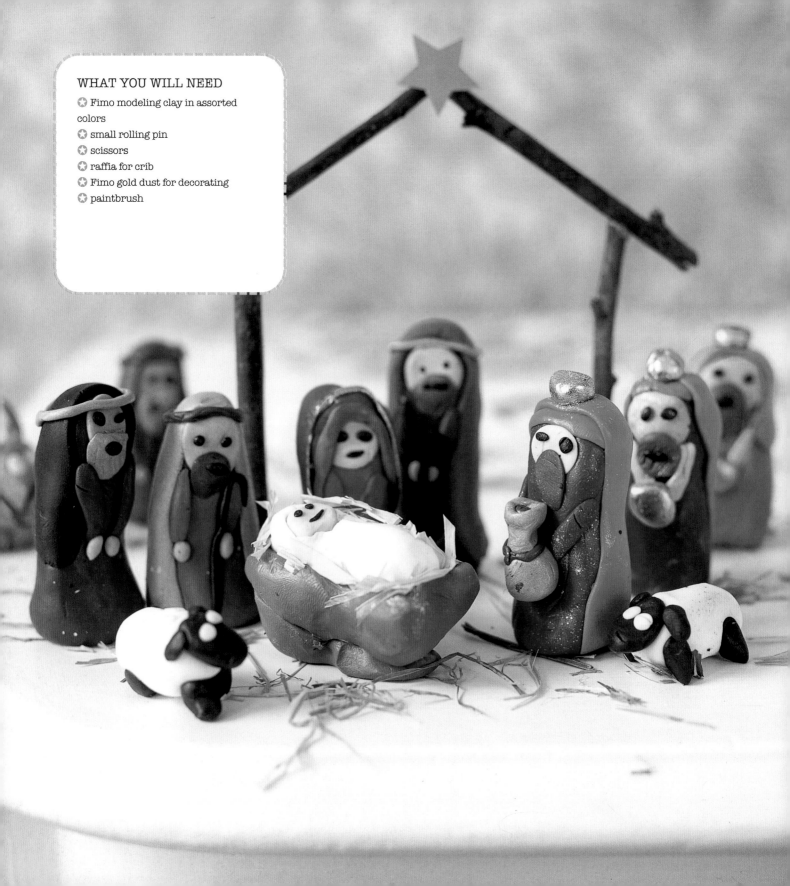

WHAT YOU WILL NEED

✪ Fimo modeling clay in assorted colors
✪ small rolling pin
✪ scissors
✪ raffia for crib
✪ Fimo gold dust for decorating
✪ paintbrush

nativity scene

A wonderful family keepsake that can be brought out every year, this nativity scene is made from Fimo colored modeling clay. Each figure is based on a simple tube shape and decorated with touches of gold.

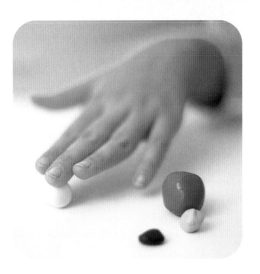

1 **MAKE BABY** Take some white modeling clay and roll out a tube shape about 1¼in/3cm in length for the baby's body. If the clay is hard, work it between the hands first to soften it, so it is easier to mold it into shape.

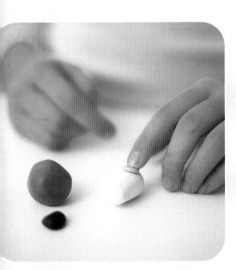

2 **MAKE FACE** Take a small piece of flesh-colored clay and roll it into a ball. Flatten it with your fingers to form a small round disc. Press the disc firmly onto the top of the body shape. Use tiny pieces of black clay to make the eyes and a mouth, and press them into position on the face.

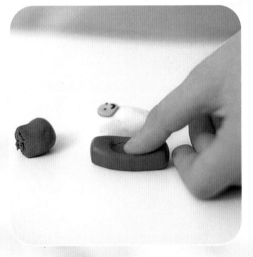

3 **MAKE CRIB** Take the brown modeling clay and roll it into a tube shape measuring about 2in/5cm in length and about 1in/2cm in diameter. Use your thumb to press down and make an indentation in the crib. Roll two balls of brown clay and press them flat to make the legs of the crib.

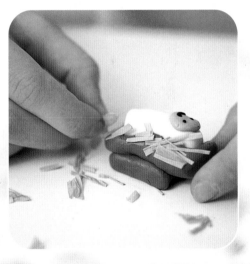

4 **DECORATE WITH RAFFIA** Use scissors to snip small pieces of raffia for the straw in the crib. Press the pieces of raffia firmly against the sides of the crib until they stick in place.

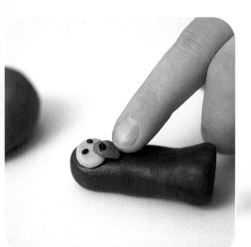

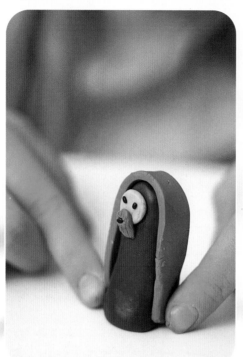

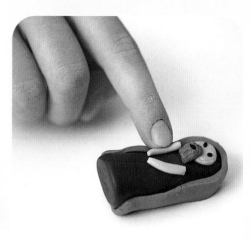

7 ATTACH ARMS
Make two small rolls of flesh-colored clay for the arms and press them firmly against the front of the body. Use more small pieces of clay to form the gifts for the kings to carry, and press them into position between the arms at the front of the body.

5 MAKE MORE FIGURES
Each figure is made from a basic tube shape formed from clay and measuring approximately 2in/5cm in length and 1in/2cm in diameter. Then take a small piece of flesh-colored clay, roll it into a ball, and press it flat to form a round disc for the face. Using the same method, make a beard from brown clay and use tiny pieces of black clay for the eyes and mouth.

6 MAKE CLOAK
To make the cloak, roll out a piece of clay to approximately 4in/10cm long by ½in/1cm wide. Fold it over the body and press firmly in place. If the cloak is too long, trim with scissors.

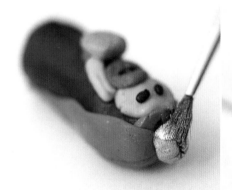

8 FINISHING
The kings' gifts and crowns are finished off with fine gold dust applied with a paintbrush. Lay the figure on its side while you apply the dust, to prevent it from falling onto the rest of the figure.

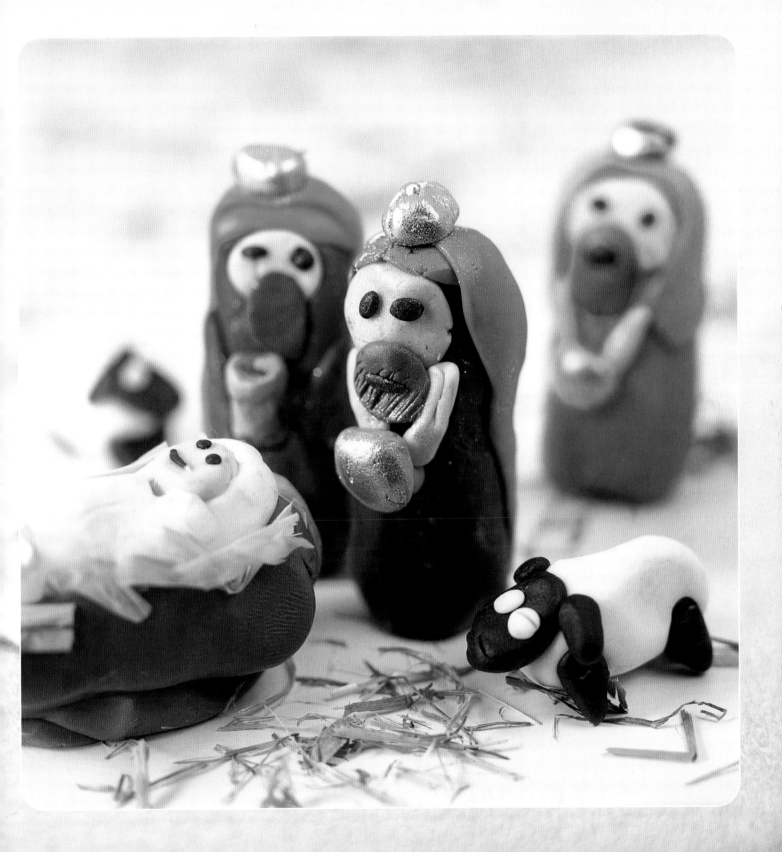

orange pomanders

These traditional scented pomanders made from oranges and decorated with cloves have been associated with Christmas since medieval times. Their sweetly spicy smell makes them welcome gifts for family and friends, but they are also pretty decorations to hang in the home or can be used to scent your closets.

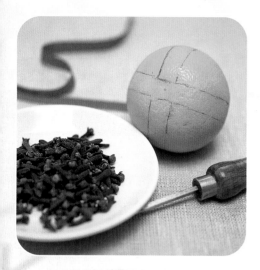

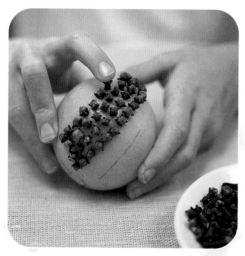

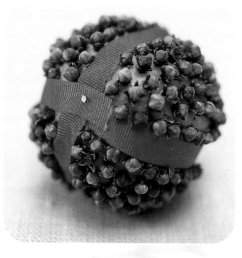

1 MARK RIBBON POSITIONS
Use the ballpoint pen to mark out the ribbon positions around the orange. (The ribbon is wrapped round the orange in the shape of a cross.) Use the awl to pierce holes for the cloves on the four quarters of the orange. Awls are very sharp, so it is advisable that an adult pierces the holes.

2 INSERT CLOVES Carefully push the cloves into the orange. The tops of the cloves can be quite brittle, so push them in gently. Continue to push the cloves into the orange until all four quarters are covered.

3 FIX RIBBON Wrap a length of ribbon around the orange so the ends overlap at the bottom of the orange. Cut the ribbon and hold the first piece in place as you wrap another length around the orange. Trim any trailing ribbon ends. Now push a pin through the ends of the ribbon to hold it securely in place.

WHAT YOU WILL NEED

- ✿ ballpoint pen
- ✿ large orange
- ✿ awl (for piercing holes)
- ✿ cloves
- ✿ 24in/60cm ribbon (½in/1cm wide)
- ✿ scissors
- ✿ pin

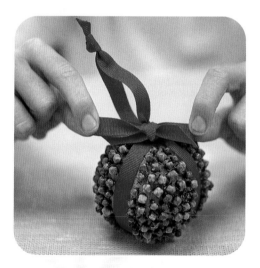

4 FINISHING Thread a length of ribbon through the top of the crossed ribbon on the orange and tie the ends together. Tie a knot in the ribbon about 2in/5cm from the top of the orange to form a loop. Now thread a further length of ribbon through the top of the ribbon and tie into a pretty bow to finish.

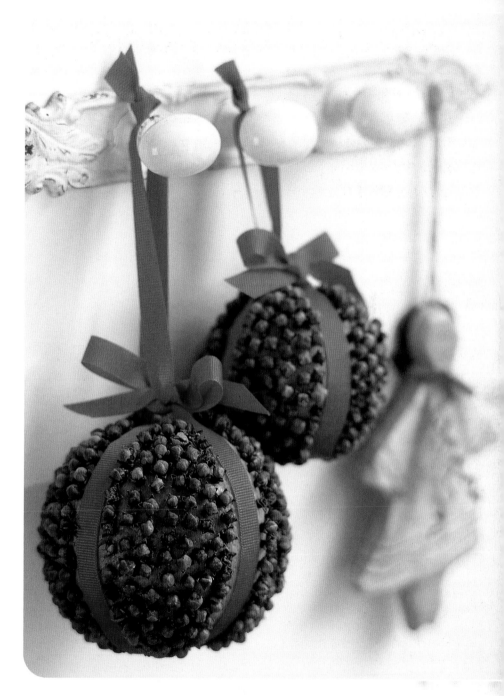

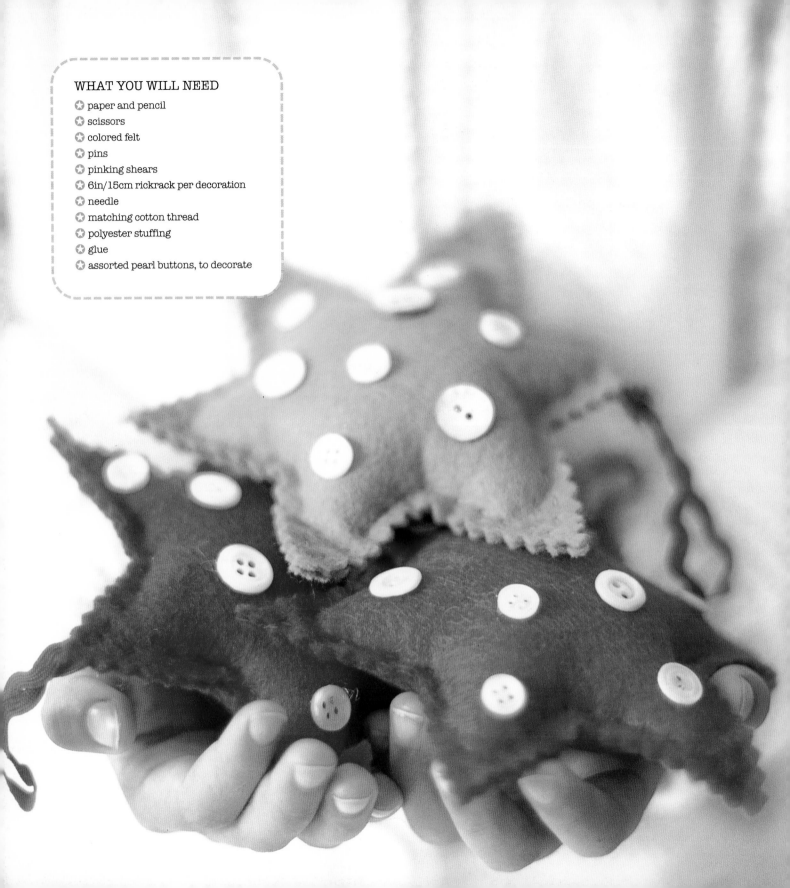

WHAT YOU WILL NEED

- ✪ paper and pencil
- ✪ scissors
- ✪ colored felt
- ✪ pins
- ✪ pinking shears
- ✪ 6in/15cm rickrack per decoration
- ✪ needle
- ✪ matching cotton thread
- ✪ polyester stuffing
- ✪ glue
- ✪ assorted pearl buttons, to decorate

hanging felt stars

Cut from red and green felt using pinking shears, these jolly tree decorations are an ideal easy sewing project for little fingers. We decorated the star shapes with pretty buttons and hung them from rickrack loops.

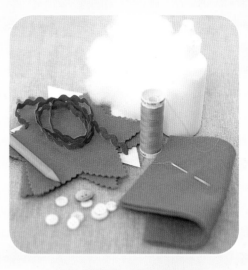

1 MAKE TEMPLATE Trace the star template on page 152 onto a piece of paper and cut it out.

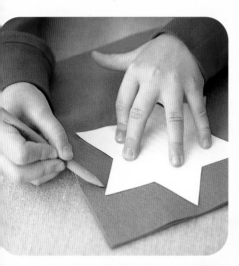

2 DRAW AROUND TEMPLATE Fold the felt in half, as you will need two star shapes per decoration. Use a pencil to draw around the star motif on the felt fabric (it may be easier if you first pin the star motif to the felt to keep it in place).

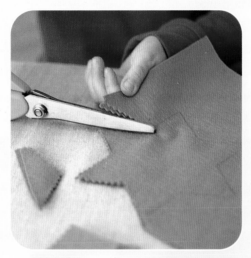

3 CUT OUT Using pinking shears, carefully cut all the way around the star shape, making sure you are cutting through both layers of fabric. The pinking shears give a zigzag effect to the edges and, if you are using cotton or linen, will prevent the fabric from fraying. If you are making more than one star decoration, it is a good idea to cut them all out at one time.

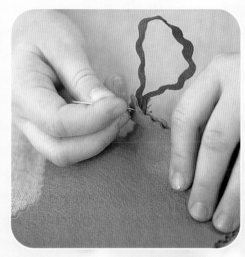

4 ATTACH LOOP Fold a 6in/15cm length of rickrack in half and place between the two layers of felt at the top of one of the points. Thread the needle. Push the needle through the two layers of felt, sandwiching the loop between them, and make two or three stitches to secure the hanging loop.

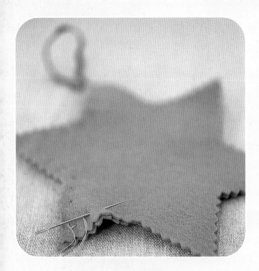

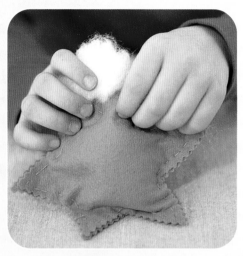

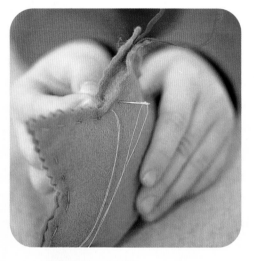

5 STITCH TOGETHER Continue stitching all the way around the points of the star, using small running stitches about ¼in/5mm from the edge. Stitch around five sides of the star, but leave the sixth side open for the stuffing.

6 STUFF HEART Carefully push the stuffing into the opening. You may need to use the end of a knitting needle or a pencil to make sure that the stuffing is right down inside all the points of the star.

7 STITCH OPENING CLOSED Hold the two layers of felt together and stitch the opening closed, again using small running stitches ¼in/5mm from the edges of the fabric. Cast off the stitching by making two or three stitches together, and snip the loose ends of the cotton.

8 FINISHING Use neat dabs of glue to stick the buttons to the front of the star decoration, then leave to dry completely. You may wish to glue buttons to the other side of the decoration (you will need extra buttons for this).

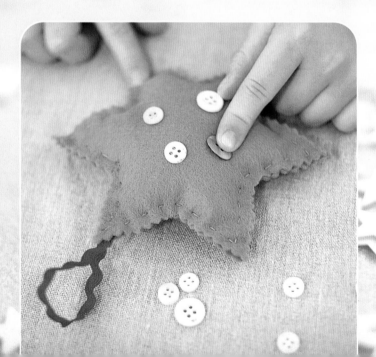

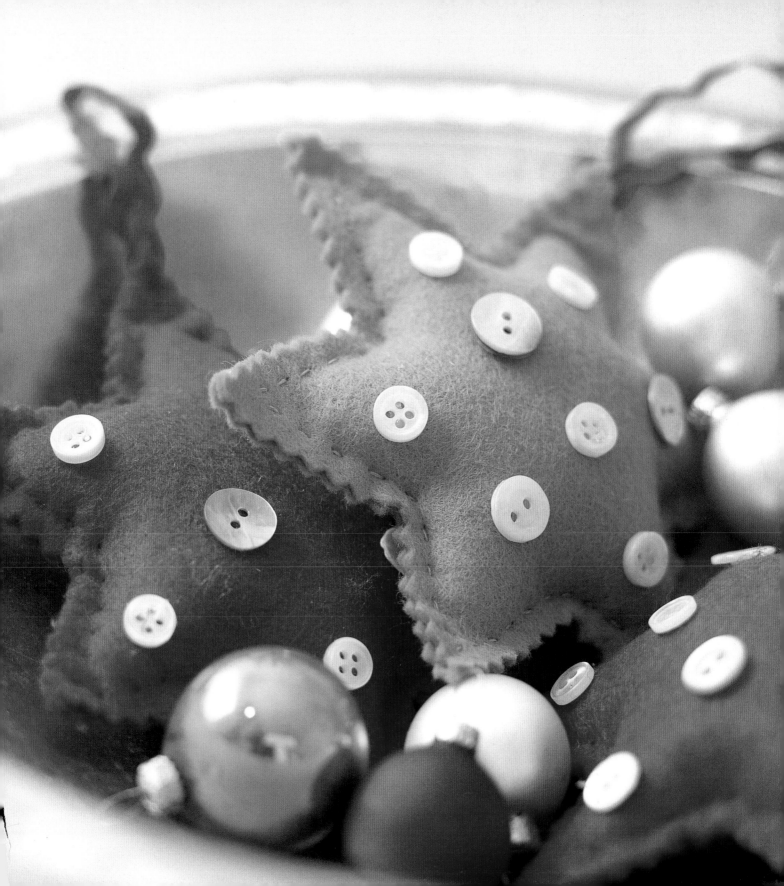

chocolate brownies

These delicious chocolate brownies are given a festive touch with pretty Christmas-tree motifs made using a stencil and sifted confectioner's sugar. If you can resist the temptation of eating them yourself, they make great gifts for teachers, family, and friends.

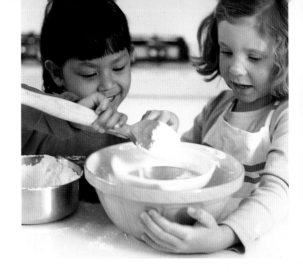

1 MIX INGREDIENTS Preheat the oven to 325°F/160°C. Cut a 10in/25cm square of foil and use it to line the base and sides of the pan. Melt the butter in a saucepan over a low heat. Crack the eggs into a mixing bowl. Pour in the sugar, then add the vanilla. Stir well with a wooden spoon. Pour in the melted butter and stir. Set a strainer over the mixing bowl and sift the cocoa and flour onto the egg mixture. Stir well.

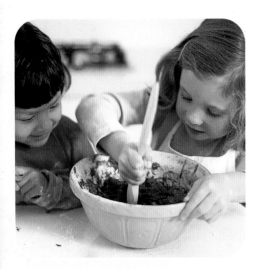

2 ADD CHOCOLATE Break the chocolate into small chunks and add to the bowl. Stir until just mixed, then spoon the mixture into the foil-lined pan. Ask an adult to help you put the pan into the oven. The brownies will take about 40 minutes to cook in the center of the oven. To test if they are ready, push a cocktail stick into one, then pull it out. If the stick is clean, they are ready; if it's sticky, leave them for another 5 minutes.

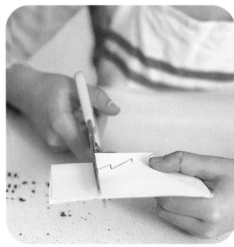

3 CUT OUT STENCIL Ask an adult to remove the pan from the oven, as it will be very hot. Leave the pan to cool on a wire rack. When completely cold, remove the brownies from the pan, peel off the foil and cut into 16 squares. Trace the Christmas tree stencil on page 155 on paper and cut out the tree shape. This is your stencil.

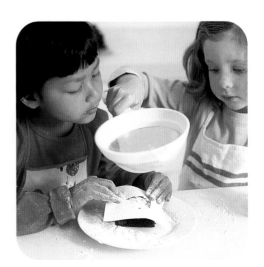

4 FINISHING Place the stencil on top of a brownie and sift confectioner's sugar over it. Carefully remove the stencil to reveal the Christmas tree motif. Repeat until all the brownies are decorated.

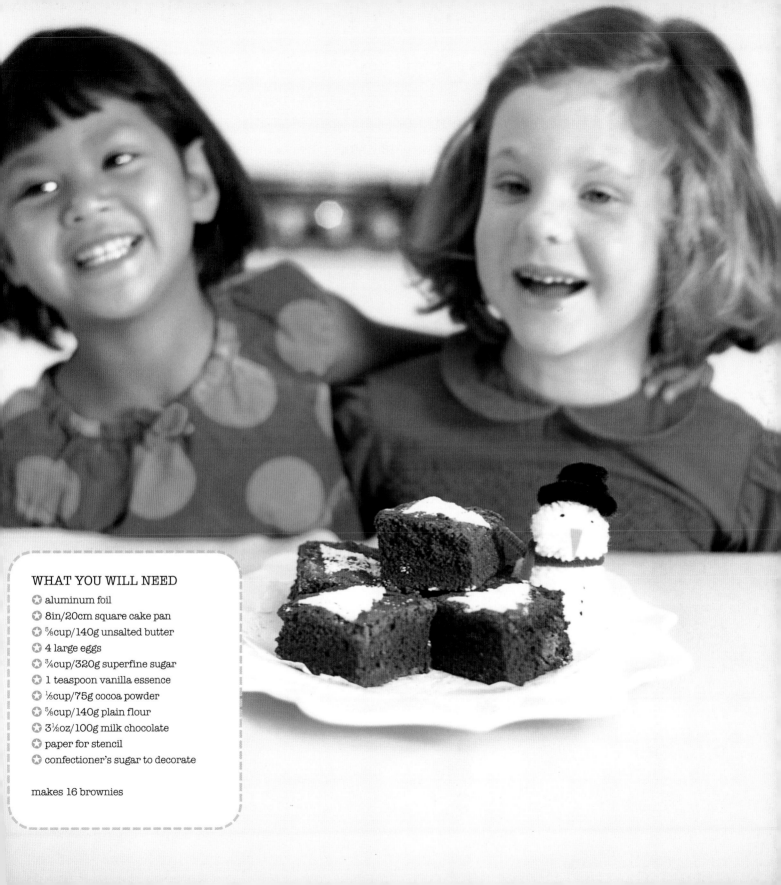

WHAT YOU WILL NEED

- ✪ aluminum foil
- ✪ 8in/20cm square cake pan
- ✪ ⅝cup/140g unsalted butter
- ✪ 4 large eggs
- ✪ ¾cup/320g superfine sugar
- ✪ 1 teaspoon vanilla essence
- ✪ ⅓cup/75g cocoa powder
- ✪ ⅝cup/140g plain flour
- ✪ 3½oz/100g milk chocolate
- ✪ paper for stencil
- ✪ confectioner's sugar to decorate

makes 16 brownies

angel tree topper

Decorate simple cones of card with a sprinkling of sparkling glitter
and a pompom to create these pretty tree-top angels complete with
a pipe-cleaner halo and wings. Quick, easy, and effective!

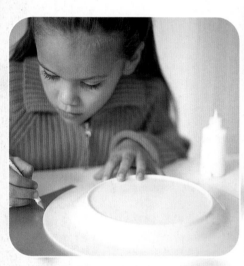

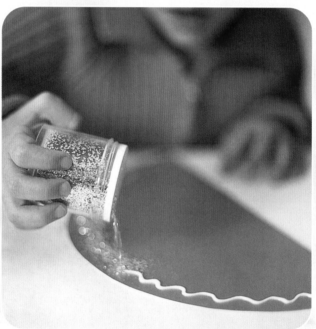

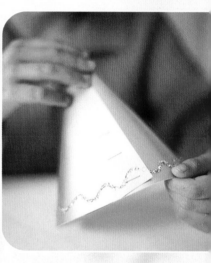

1 DRAW AROUND PLATE
Place the plate on the silver card stock
and draw around half of it to create a
semi-circle for the cone. Cut out.

2 APPLY GLITTER Use glue to draw a
scalloped line all around the curved edge of the
semicircular piece of card. Sprinkle silver glitter
generously over the glue and leave for a few
minutes. Shake off any excess glitter and allow
the glue to dry completely.

3 FORM CONE SHAPE Form the
card semicircle into a cone shape (folding
it gently in half and making a slight crease
at the center of the card makes it a bit
easier to form a cone). Use a stapler to join
the edges of the card.

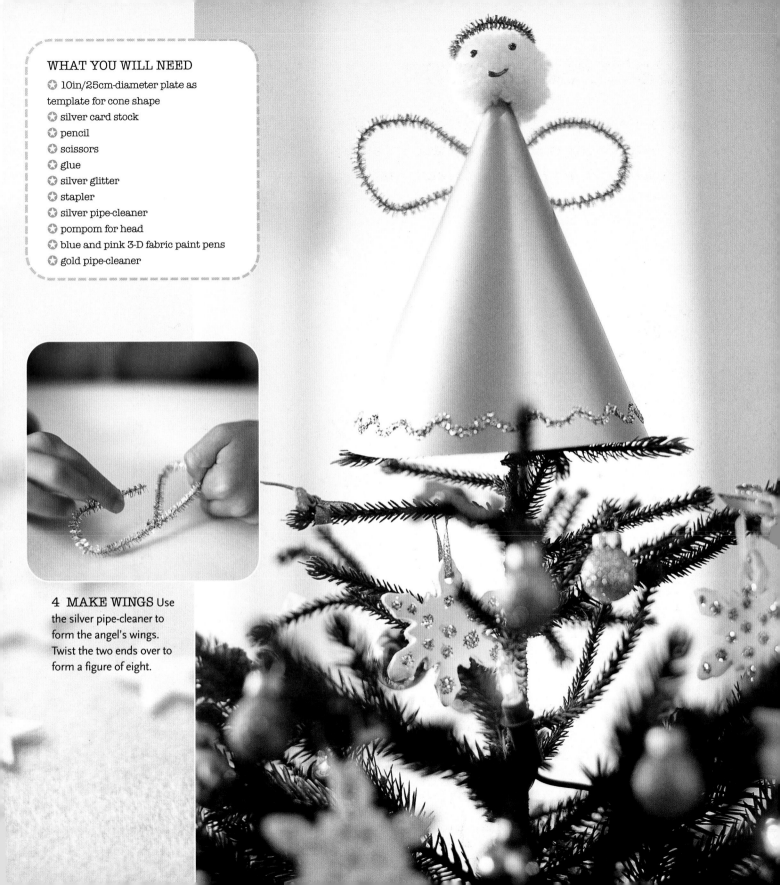

WHAT YOU WILL NEED

- 10in/25cm-diameter plate as template for cone shape
- silver card stock
- pencil
- scissors
- glue
- silver glitter
- stapler
- silver pipe-cleaner
- pompom for head
- blue and pink 3-D fabric paint pens
- gold pipe-cleaner

4 MAKE WINGS Use the silver pipe-cleaner to form the angel's wings. Twist the two ends over to form a figure of eight.

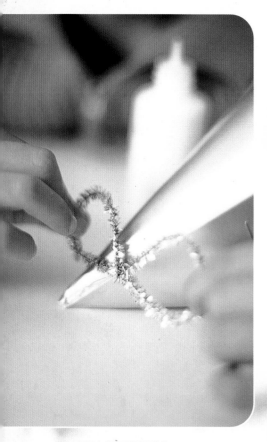

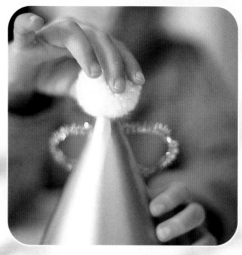

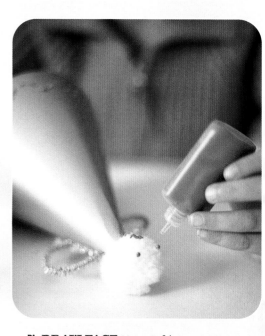

5 ATTACH WINGS Apply a dab of glue to the center of the wings and glue them to the back of the cone, about 2in/5cm down from the top. Allow glue to dry completely.

6 GLUE ON POMPOM HEAD Either use a ready-made pompom or make your own following the instructions on pages 28–29. Glue the pompom to the top of the cone and leave to dry.

7 DRAW FACE Use 3-D fabric paint pens in pink and blue to carefully draw the angel's eyes and mouth onto the pompom. Leave to dry.

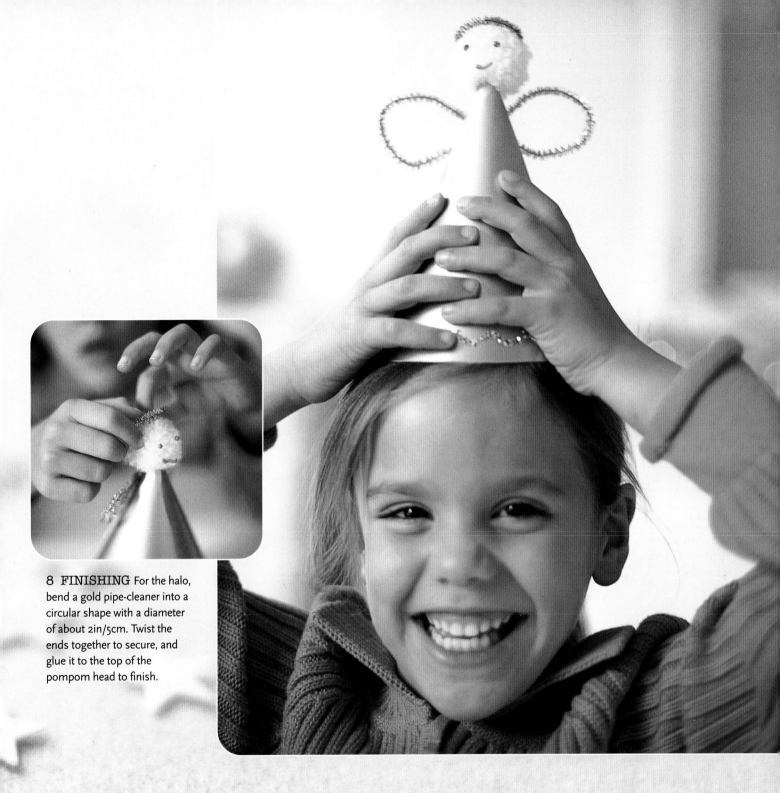

8 FINISHING For the halo, bend a gold pipe-cleaner into a circular shape with a diameter of about 2in/5cm. Twist the ends together to secure, and glue it to the top of the pompom head to finish.

christmas stocking

Create this pretty Shaker-style stocking in cream wool and decorate with a simple heart motif and a mother-of-pearl button. You could even make one for each member of the family and tie on name tags.

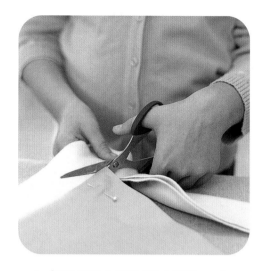

1 CREATE A TEMPLATE Trace the stocking template on page 155 onto a piece of paper. Now enlarge it on a photocopier at 200 percent to make it the right size. Cut out the template. Fold the cream wool fabric in half and pin the template to the fabric. Cut out the stocking pieces.

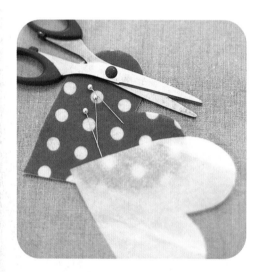

2 CUT OUT HEART MOTIF Trace the heart template on page 155 onto a piece of paper and cut it out. Pin the template to the felt and cut out a heart shape to decorate the front of the stocking.

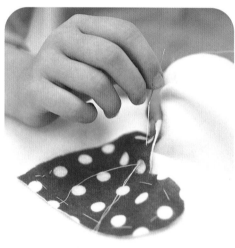

3 BASTE HEART TO STOCKING Thread the needle with white cotton and baste the heart to the front stocking piece.

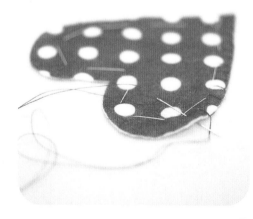

4 BLANKET-STITCH HEART Now thread the needle with red cotton and work small blanket stitches all the way around the heart motif. When you have finished, carefully remove the basting. Now use a dab of glue to stick the pearl button to the very center of the heart.

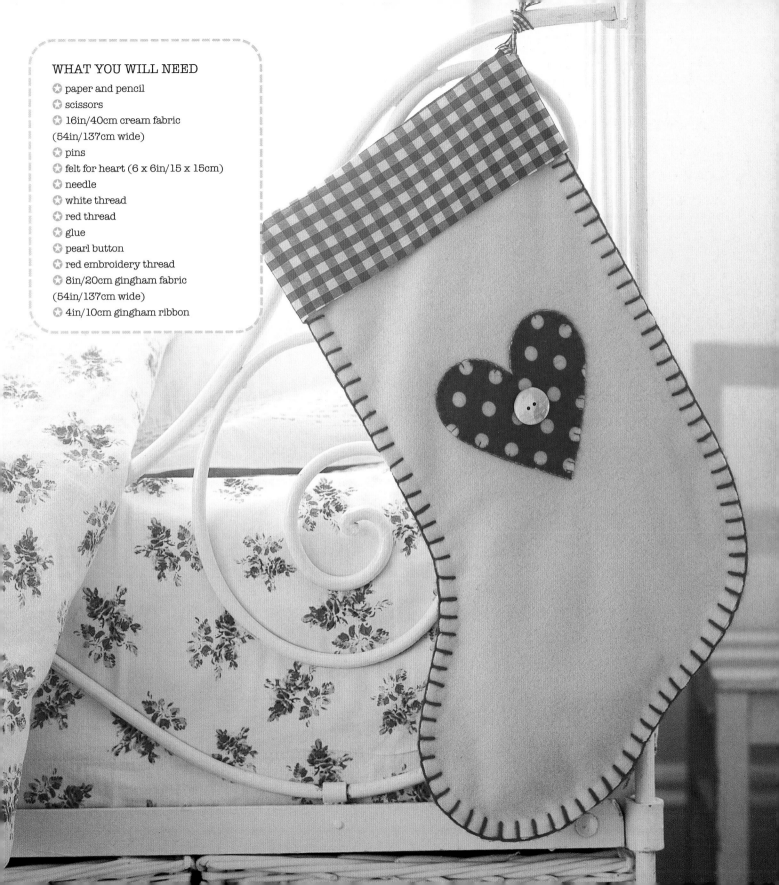

WHAT YOU WILL NEED

- ✪ paper and pencil
- ✪ scissors
- ✪ 16in/40cm cream fabric
  (54in/137cm wide)
- ✪ pins
- ✪ felt for heart (6 x 6in/15 x 15cm)
- ✪ needle
- ✪ white thread
- ✪ red thread
- ✪ glue
- ✪ pearl button
- ✪ red embroidery thread
- ✪ 8in/20cm gingham fabric
  (54in/137cm wide)
- ✪ 4in/10cm gingham ribbon

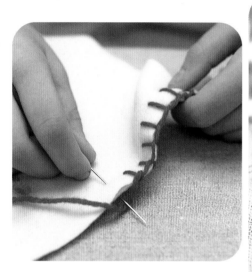

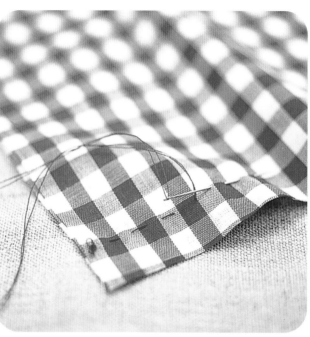

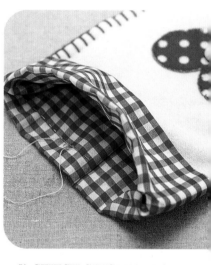

5 STITCH STOCKING TOGETHER With right sides facing, baste the two stocking pieces together. Turn right side out. Thread a needle with the red embroidery thread and work blanket stitch all the way around the edges of the stocking, leaving the top edges open. Press flat with an iron (it is advisable for an adult to do this).

6 MAKE GINGHAM BORDER Take the piece of gingham fabric. Fold it in half lengthwise, with right sides together, and stitch the side seams together using small running stitches. Turn right side out and press flat with an iron (it is advisable for an adult to do this).

7 STITCH GINGHAM TO STOCKING Turn a ½in/1cm hem to the inside of the gingham and press flat. Tuck about 3in/8cm of the gingham fabric inside the stocking and fold the remainder of the fabric over the top of the stocking, with the hemmed edge on the outside. Sew small running stitches all around the top of the gingham fabric to hold it in place.

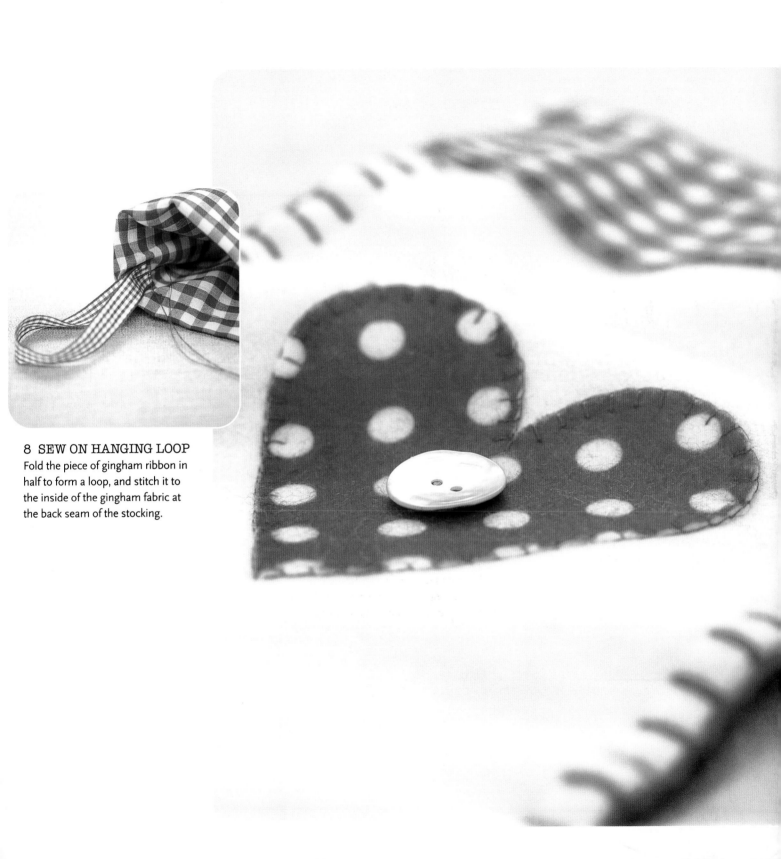

8 SEW ON HANGING LOOP
Fold the piece of gingham ribbon in half to form a loop, and stitch it to the inside of the gingham fabric at the back seam of the stocking.

templates

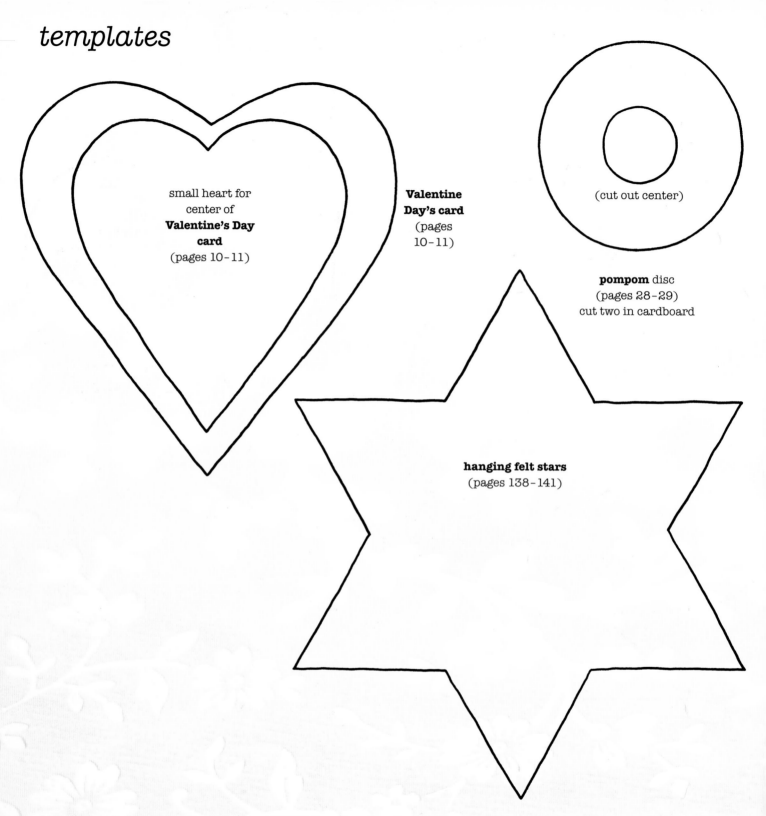

small heart for
center of
**Valentine's Day
card**
(pages 10-11)

**Valentine
Day's card**
(pages
10-11)

(cut out center)

pompom disc
(pages 28-29)
cut two in cardboard

hanging felt stars
(pages 138-141)

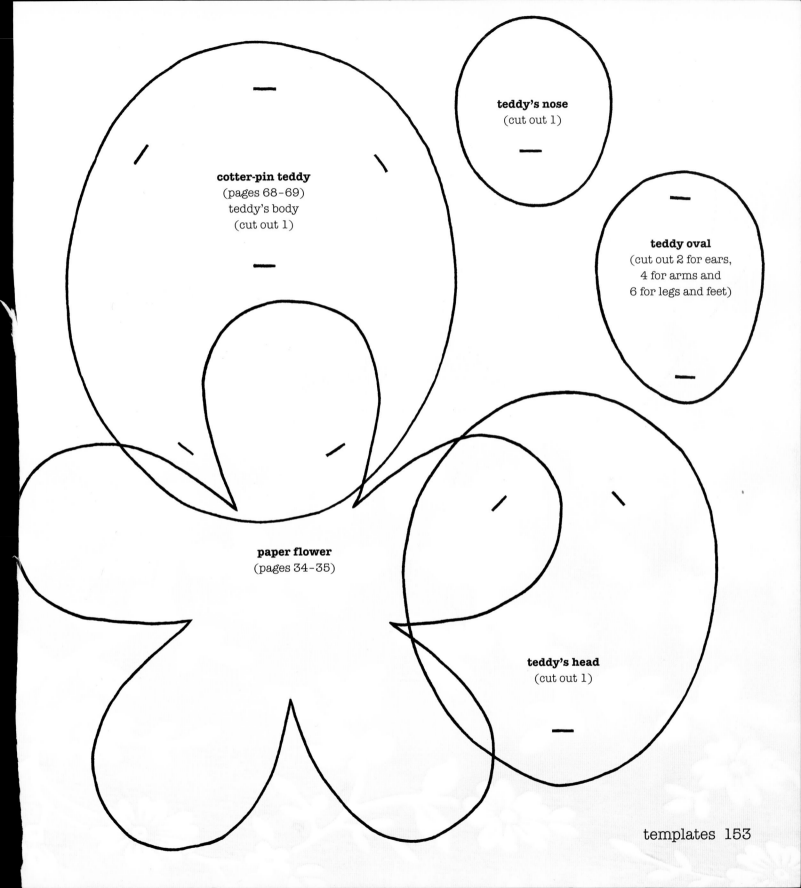

teddy's nose
(cut out 1)

cotter-pin teddy
(pages 68–69)
teddy's body
(cut out 1)

teddy oval
(cut out 2 for ears,
4 for arms and
6 for legs and feet)

paper flower
(pages 34–35)

teddy's head
(cut out 1)

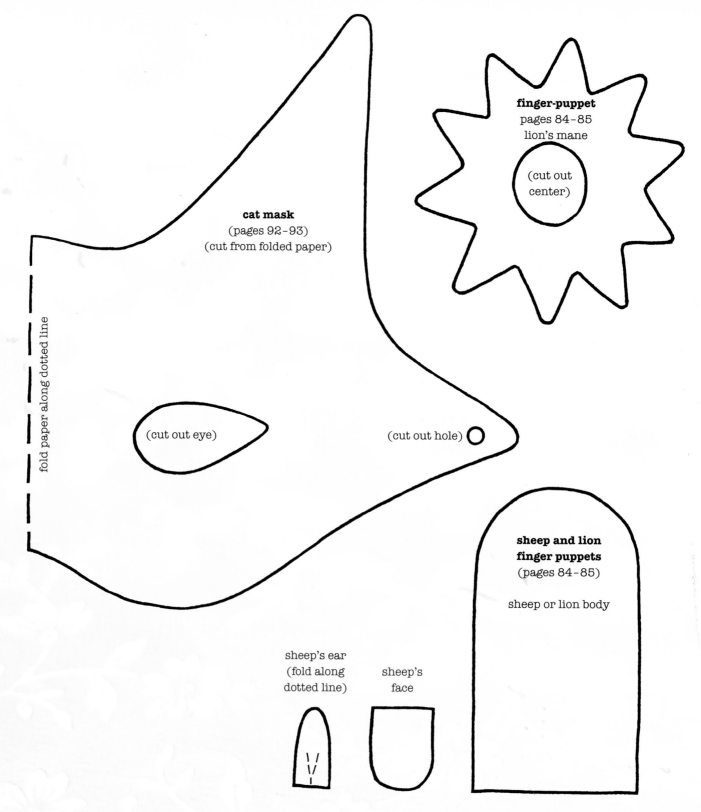

finger-puppet
pages 84–85
lion's mane

(cut out center)

cat mask
(pages 92–93)
(cut from folded paper)

fold paper along dotted line

(cut out eye)

(cut out hole) ○

**sheep and lion
finger puppets**
(pages 84–85)

sheep or lion body

sheep's ear
(fold along
dotted line)

sheep's
face

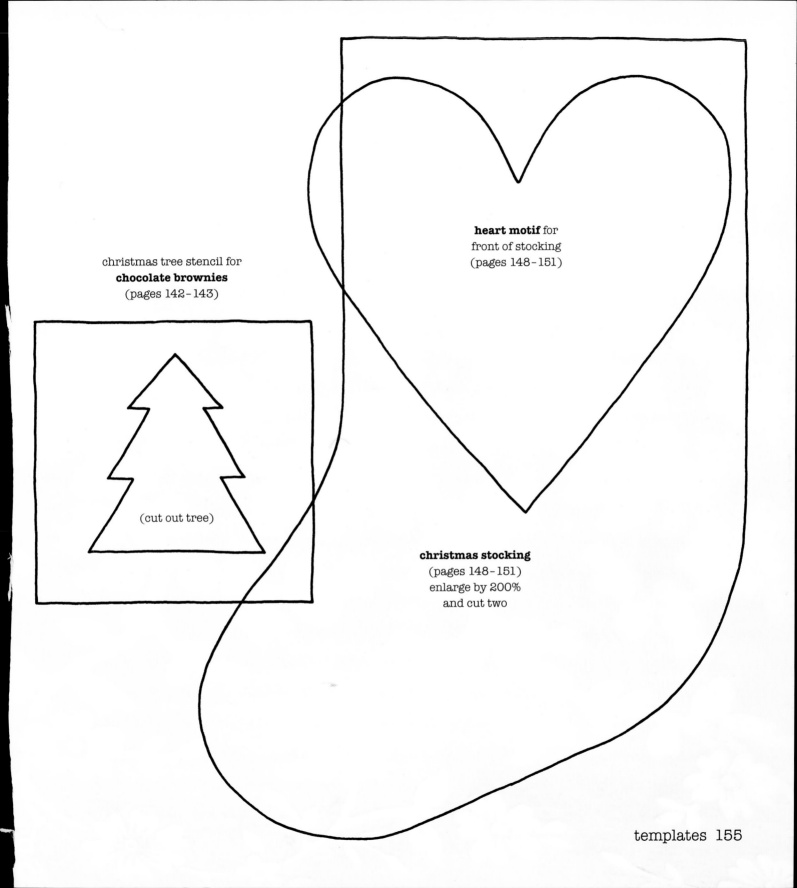

christmas tree stencil for
chocolate brownies
(pages 142–143)

(cut out tree)

heart motif for
front of stocking
(pages 148–151)

christmas stocking
(pages 148–151)
enlarge by 200%
and cut two

templates 155

sources

CRAFTING SUPPLIES

A. C. MOORE
www.acmoore.com
Craft superstores carrying modeling clay, tealights, pipe-cleaners, and stencils.

DICK BLICK
www.dickblick.com
Cardmaking supplies, crepe, tissue, and decorative paper, stencils, ribbon, and more.

BRITEX FABRICS
146 Geary Street
San Francisco, CA 94108
415-392-2910
www.britexfabrics.com
Ribbons, trims, and notions.

THE BUTTON EMPORIUM & RIBBONRY
914 S.W. 11th Avenue
Portland, OR 97205
503-228-6372
www.buttonemporium.com
Vintage and assorted decorative buttons.

HYMAN HENDLER & SONS
67 West 38th Street
New York, NY 10018
212-840-8393
www.hymanhendler.com
Novelty and vintage ribbons.

IKEA
www.ikea.com
Unpainted wooden photo frames, plain tins for découpaging, and cute accessories.

JOANN FABRICS
Locations nationwide
Visit *www.joann.com* for details of your nearest store.
A wide selection of paper, card, fabric, scrapbooking materials, and more.

KARI ME AWAY
www.karimeaway.com
Rickrack trim in a large variety of colors. Also cute novelty buttons in different shapes, and glass beads.

KATE'S PAPERIE
561 Broadway
New York, NY 10012
212-941-9816
888-809-9880
www.katespaperie.com
Rubber stamps for kids.

LOOSE ENDS
2065 Madrona Ave SE
Salem, OR 97302
503-390-7457
www.looseends.com
Paper for découpage, ribbon, ties, and trims.

MICHAELS
www.michaels.com
Every kind of art and craft material, including air-drying modeling clay, stamps, ink pads, embellishments, paints, and glues.

M&J TRIMMING
www.mjtrim.com
Fancy trims, including rhinestones, sequined flowers, ribbons, rickrack, and beaded braid.

PAPER CREATIONS
www.papercreations.com
Supplies for papercrafting and scrapbooking as well as rubber stamps.

PAPER SOURCE
1-888-PAPER-11
www.paper-source.com
Envelopes, blank cards, and handmade paper, as well as crafting basics.

PAPER WISHES
888-300-3406
www.paperwishes.com
Paper, scrapbooks, stamping accessories, stickers, tools, and more.

PEARL ART AND CRAFTS SUPPLIES
1-800-451-7327
www.pearlpaint.com
Brushes, modeling clay, glue, paper, and card.

PRIZM
The Artist's Supply Store
5688 Mayfield Rd.
Cleveland, OH 44124
www.prizmart.com
Paints, paper, brushes, and more.

TARGET
www.target.com
Paper, tools, and more.

TINSEL TRADING CO.
47 West 38th Street
New York, NY 10018
212-730-1030
www.tinseltrading.com
Vintage buttons, beads, and ribbons.

UTRECHT
www.utrechtart.com
Modeling clay, natural wooden frames,
paints, and craft paper.

BAKING SUPPLIES

THE BAKERS KITCHEN
419-381-9693
www.thebakerskitchen.net
Cake decorating and baking, including
cookie cutters in novel shapes.

CANDYLAND CRAFTS
201 W. Main Street
Somerville, NJ 08876
908-685-0410
www.candylandcrafts.com
Cookie cutters and piping gel.

NEW YORK CAKE SUPPLIES
56 West 22nd Street
New York, NY 10010
800-942-2539
www.nycake.com
Sugar paste, edible decorations, food colors,
flavorings, and cookie cutters in every shape.

GARDEN SUPPLIES

AVANT GARDENS
710 High Hill Road
North Dartmouth, MA 02747
508-998-8819
www.avantgardensne.com
Alpine plants and colorful annuals.

E BURLAP
877-885-7527
www.eburlap.com
Burlap rolls and squares for general garden
tasks as well as the burlap tote project.

GARDENER'S SUPPLY COMPANY
1-888-833-1412
www.gardeners.com
Everything for the garden, from tools to
pottery to fertilizers and soil to plant
markers.

HOME DEPOT
www.homedepot.com
Visit one of their 1500 stores for garden tools
and equipment, and potting mixes.

HOUSE FABRIC
314-968-0090
www.housefabric.com
Burlap and canvas fabrics and printed cotton
fabrics ideal for the lavender bags project.

LOWE'S HOME CENTERS
www.lowes.com
Soil, sand, potting mix, and garden tools.

MERRIT LAVENDER FARM
87450 McTimmons Lane
Bandon, OR 97411
541-347-7190
www.lavenderladyfarm.com
Dried lavender for lavender bags.

MT TAHOMA NURSERY
253-847-9827
www.backyardgardener.com
Rock garden and alpine plants.

THE NATIONAL GARDENING
ASSOCIATION
Visit their website for kids at
www.kidsgardening.com
Their "Gardening with Kids" store
www.kidsgardeningstore.com offers mini
wheelbarrows, gloves, kids' tools, plant
markers, a garden tool organizer and more.

NICHOLS GARDEN NURSERY
1190 Old Salem Road NE
Albany, OR 97321
1-800-422-3985
www.nicholsgardennursery.com
Every kind of vegetable seed imaginable,
including many unusual heirloom varieties.

SMITH & HAWKEN
1-800-940-1170
www.smithandhawken.com
Their "Sprouts" line offers watering cans,
trugs, pint-sized tool kits, and other
essentials for green-thumbed kids.

picture credits

PHOTOGRAPHY

VANESSA DAVIES

Pages 1–6, 10–11, 12–13, 14–15, 16–17, 18 background, 20–21, 26–27, 28–29, 32–33, 34–35, 40–41, 46–47, 49, 50–51, 52–53, 54–55, 58–59, 64–65, 68–69, 72–73, 80–81, 84–85, 86–87, 92–93, 94–95, 96–97, 116–117, 118–119, 128–129

POLLY WREFORD

Pages 4 background, 7 background, 8, 9, 10–11 background, 12–13 background, 18–19, 22–25, 30–31, 32–33 background, 36–39, 42–45, 48, 50–51 background, 52–53 background, 56–57, 60–61, 62–63, 66–67, 70–71, 72–73 background, 74–75, 76–77, 78–79, 80–81 background, 82–83, 86–87 background, 88–89, 90–91, 92–93 background, 96–97 background, 98–99, 100–101, 102–103, 104–105, 106–107, 108–109, 110–111, 112–113, 114–115, 120–121, 122–123, 124–125, 126–127, 130–131, 132–135, 136–137, 138–141, 142–143, 144–147, 148–151

index

acknowledgments

Thanks to the Norfolk Lavender Company for supplying the lavender, to J. Arthur Bowers for the potting mix used in the gardening projects, and to Hobbycraft for supplying a wonderful selection of paper, fabrics, ribbons, and other items for many of the projects.

Thank you also to the models who appear in the photographs in this book, including Ahana, Aimee, Alessandra, Alissia and Saskia, Anna and Jessica, Archie and Ollie, Archie, Arthur, Asha, Cameron, Chanelle and Ayeisha, Ella and Ivo, Ella, Eva, Eve, Georgia, Gus and Kit, Harriet, Havana and Hassia, Jack and Gabriella, Jack, Jessica, Jordan, Kaan, Katie, Lilee, Louis, Millie, Olivia, Oscar, Tabitha, Tahiti, and William and James.

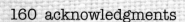